Childfree and Sterilized

Childfree and Sterilized

Women's Decisions and Medical Responses

Annily Campbell

CASSELL

London and New York

Cassell
Wellington House, 125 Strand, London WC2R 0BB
370 Lexington Avenue, New York, NY 10017-6550

First published 1999

British Library Cataloguing-in-Publication Data
A catalogue record for this book is available from the British Library.
ISBN 0 304 33746 3 Hardback
       0 304 33747 1 Paperback

Library of Congress Cataloging-in-Publication Data
Campbell, Annily, 1947–
   Childfree and sterilized : women's decisions and medical responses
Annily Campbell.
       p. cm.
   Includes bibliographical references and index.
   ISBN 0-304-33746-3.—ISBN 0-304-33747-1 (pbk.)
   1. Sterilization of women—Psychological aspects.
   2. Sterilization of women—Social aspects—Great Britain.
   3. Sterilization (Birth control)—Psychological aspects.
   4. Childlessness—Psychological aspects.   5. Childlessness—Social
aspects—Great Britain.   6. Women—Psychology.   I. Title.
RG138.C35 1999   99-18201
618. 1—dc21   CIP

Typeset by York House Typographic Ltd, London
Printed and bound in Great Britain by Biddles Ltd, Guildford and
King's Lynn

For my mother and my father,
Mary McNeill and John George Ashe

Contents

Acknowledgements

When I telephoned and wrote to the women participants of this book to check details and finalize entries (an increasingly frantic occurrence in the final month), I often heard them expressing their thanks to me. I found this disconcerting as I felt that I should be thanking them for telling their stories for the book. First and greatest thanks, then, go to the 23 women in this study who had 'always known' that they did not want children and so, desiring neither pregnancy nor motherhood, decided that sterilization would free them from monthly panics and scares as well as the necessity of continuing to use other methods of contraception. Thanks also to Jane, whose contribution as a woman who thought deeply about her decision to have a child when she was older was a valuable addition to the research, and provided an excellent contrast to women who were sure that they did not want children.

Chris Eilbeck allowed her prose to be used in addition to the diary entries, Emma kept a personal diary from which she has allowed me to use extracts and Jude provided a reflective and insightful account of her perceptions of the process of being interviewed. Professor Simon Conway Morris gave permission for me to quote from his opening address to the audience at the 1996 Royal Institution Christmas Lectures series and Jacky Fleming has allowed me to refer to her cartoons which provide sharp comment on so many aspects of women's lives.

I am indebted to a number of consultants, doctors, GPs and family planning professionals for their time and patience in providing answers to questions. Professor Lord Robert Winston (Institute of Obstetrics and Gynaecology, Hammersmith Hospital) took time to respond to several letters and queries about the incidence of sterilization reversals on child-free women. Professor John Newton (Birmingham Women's Hospital) provided an academic paper which proved invaluable for showing that childfree women were not taken seriously when they applied to be sterilized. Mr Robert Sawer and Mr John Pogmore (both Birmingham Women's Hospital and The Priory Hospital, Birmingham) were generous with time for interviews and phone calls. Tricia Newton (a nurse-specialist in family planning) and Dr Pat Plant (Senior Clinical Medical Officer; both at Handsworth Family Planning and Community Centre, Birmingham) shared much information from their extensive experience and work with women. Ann Dorow provided insights into the history and current practice of Birmingham Brook Advisory Centre.

Terry Lovell, my supervisor at the University of Warwick, enabled me to widen my perspective and to make links with global considerations of contraception and birth control, and the nature of choice and decision-making. She was challenging and vigorous when she spotted my own prejudices and the need to prove my own points although, of course, I continue to be totally responsible for further examples which have crept into the book despite her comments. Thanks also for encouragement and direction pointers from Dr Richard Lampard, also at the University of Warwick. Dorothy Sheridan and staff provided excellent research facilities and additional information on early Mass-Observation surveys at the Mass-Observation Archive, University of Sussex in Brighton. Professor Sheila Hunt and Gayle Letherby provided positive critical feedback and many practical and insightful comments and suggestions.

Many people put up with hours of discussion and debate, and often had to endure (no doubt repetitious) rehearsal of the 'next stage' of the work. Grateful thanks, then, to my dearest friends, Margaret Hawtin, Claire Jackson and Daniele Joly, and to my colleagues and friends at the University of Derby, especially the students and the tutor-team of the Women's Studies course, for their encouragement and support and for maintaining an enthusiasm for all things feminist. I always appreciated John Dolan's wonderful 'Edmund' impressions.

This book is about childfree women but does not take a separatist stand. Women's struggle is boundaried by many ideologies, and I have always believed that the 'motherhood divide' can be a most effective separator. Thanks to all of the people who have children and who love them to bits, especially those who allow me and my partner Mike to share in their growing up: Claire and Rick, with Hannah and Becky; Daniele and Nicholas, and Gustavo who is so sorely missed; Barbara and Bob, with the talented Ruth and the very special Joe. Chris and Frank, John and Carol, with Nathan and Drew, Barry and Morag, with Miles and Jody, Susan with Brandon, are loved relatives, and parents and children in the 'new' South Africa.

Closer to home, and with the deliberate intent of causing them the greatest embarrassment. I include David and Martin, my own (now adult) children whose growing up gave me much food for thought and who are two people I wouldn't be without. My sister Anne, who for much of our lives has been so far and yet so near. Finally, my partner, Mike Poppleton, who listened (often), was supportive (unstintingly) and encouraging (always) and is the person I couldn't be without.

Preface

There have always been women without children. Women do not have children for a variety of reasons – and not only for the traditionally assumed 'she can't'. Instead, for a number of women, the reason is that 'she won't'. This book presents the stories of 23 sterilized, childfree women. Most of them insist that they had always known that they did not want to have children and all of them decided to be sterilized rather than continuing with other forms of contraception. They were so determined that their childfree choice would be reflected in their lifestyle that they considered all contraceptive options available to them, made use of some for a time, then decided on elective sterilization.

In a world where the majority of women who can, do go on to become mothers, this appears to be a normal, obvious and usually achievable goal for women. Behind much of the thinking about the state of motherhood is an often unquestioned assumption that all women who are mothers planned for and want their children, and that women who have no children want them but have 'a problem'. According to global population figures 88 per cent of women in the world will have had at least one child by the time that they have reached the age of 45, with the majority of the remaining 12 per cent eager to achieve motherhood. Yet within that 88 per cent there will be women who would have preferred to have had fewer children; others who would rather not have had children so early in their lives; and many who would have desired the opportunity to be more proactive in timing their pregnancies and the number of children born to them. There will also be a small number of women who wanted to have no children at all. Of this latter, again in global terms, only very few women will be in a position and able to act to ensure that they remain childfree. In brief, the fact that a woman has had a child is no indication of whether or not she wanted to do so.

Official abortion figures identify that there are around 75 million unplanned and unwanted pregnancies annually, of which 30 million continue to full term and 45 million are terminated (UNFPA, 1997). Many women die because of difficulties in obtaining an early, safe termination and, far from preventing or discouraging abortion, prohibitions and obstacles merely make the process even more hazardous for a determined woman. Whilst access to early abortion, therefore, is essential for comprehensive family planning (Huston, 1992) there is strong cultural disapproval of women who choose termination. Married women in particular may meet resistance from doctors 'who regard them as pathological or just plain wrong in their decision' (Richardson, 1993).

Because having a child is what most women say that they want, such a seemingly normal activity is seen as the natural order of things and there is an often expressed belief that a woman is fulfilled through motherhood, she is made whole and becomes a real woman: once woman is mother she has achieved her biological destiny. However, biology and an assumed irresistible drive towards reproduction is far from the only reason for women wanting to have children and going on to become mothers. In Britain and in America, some women are saying openly that motherhood does not attract them and that their intention is to remain without children. Increasingly, their voice is heard through the media and confirmed by research such as that conducted by the Family Policy Studies Centre, which highlights that one in five British women in the 30 plus age range have decided against having children and may never have them (McAllister, 1998). Even in its early stages that study, using national statistics, showed that many women since the 1960s were delaying or postponing having babies and that as many as one-fifth may choose to remain childfree throughout their lives (Condy, 1995).

Women determined to remain childfree must continue to monitor and thwart their body's regular, monthly impetus towards conception and pregnancy, choosing from a wide range of methods of contraception including pills, prophylactics, IUDs, creams and chemicals, and they may also resort to post-conception measures including morning-after pills and abortion. Even though using these methods of contraception, however, they continue to be potentially fertile and those who intend to remain childfree must continue to be vigilant about contraception within their heterosexual relationships. They must treat their bodies in the same way as women who plan to cease using contraception at some future point so as to have a baby, and this need to continue with contraceptive measures becomes increasingly meaningless for women who have already decided to remain childfree.

In order to gain release from an irksome responsibility, possibly to guard against pressure within a relationship for a change of mind, and given the appropriate information, a large measure of determination and sufficient amounts of money (increasingly so as the NHS becomes more budget-conscious), a small number of childfree women consider and seek sterilization as their ultimate choice of contraception. This does not always meet with success. The experience of rejection and refusal of decisions about personal reproduction was met with outrage by the women in this study, especially when the choices of other women to become mothers were accepted and unchallenged. Emma was initially furious and railed against what she experienced as patriarchal control: over a period of time, this feeling gradually gave way to a dull feeling of despair tempered with anger (see 'Emma's Story'). Jill, aged 40, was more often quietly amused at people's response, keeping her reply to herself; 'people were more hostile when I was younger, and used to ask "How can you make such a permanent decision now?" I've always been tempted to pose the same question when someone tells me they are pregnant'; and Helen, aged 38, made the point, 'I think that if a woman of 16 is able to decide to have a baby then a woman of the same age should be able to decide not to. After all, both decisions are irreversible . . .'

Whilst the age of 16 may seem too young for such a momentous decision to be made, some doctors appear to have varying opinions on what they feel they could consider as the appropriate age for a woman to be mature enough to state firmly that she does not want children and does want to be sterilized. This arbitrary age is rarely set below 25 years and is more likely considered to be when a woman is at least 30 and often when she is in her mid-thirties. The younger a woman is when she makes her first application, the more likely she is to hear, 'Go away and come back when you are married . . .' (Ann D. aged 40) and to have the experience of 'being laughed out of the surgery' (Jude, aged 31); and many of the responses in diary entries and during follow-up interviews demonstrate how common this is. Several women emphasized that the decision not to have children had been made many years before the decision to be sterilized rather than – as doctors appeared to believe – a recent and rather whimsical thought. Sally, aged 46, was aggrieved at such peculiar attitudes and felt that doctors may be guilty of illogical reasoning when they hear a woman insist that she does not want children. She illustrated what she perceived as the irrational nature of the refusals:

> If I had gone along to my GP at the age of 30 and said, 'I want a baby but I don't seem to be getting anywhere', he wouldn't have said, 'Are you old enough to know what you're doing? Do you realize it's irreversible?' . . . They don't seem to take the trouble to check out why people want to have babies because that's just considered to be normal – but they consider it odd that I don't want any, and bizarre that I've been sterilized. (Sally)

The stories told by the women who participated in this study reflect the journey which led to their opting for sterilization. Each woman describes the practical considerations and arrangements of the task, including the initial difficulties in finding a sympathetic doctor to take them seriously and refer them to a hospital which would carry out the procedure, with a consultant willing to sterilize a childfree woman. They comment on the social experience of being childfree in a world which expects women to become mothers, the consequences of refusing to continue with traditional contraceptive methods and their experiences with practitioners in the medical world.

In demanding to make their own reproductive choices these childfree women knew that they were flouting unwritten codes and expectations about the way that women should behave, and were made aware that they were breaching social conventions by disagreeing with and challenging medical pronouncements and decision-making. Far from weakening their resolve, however, they became more certain of their right to stop using other contraceptives and to opt to be sterilized. The words of Sandy, aged 36, sum up much of the determination around this issue when she stated quite firmly, 'My body – my decision . . .'.

Emma's Story: 1993–1997

Emma was 23 years old and had not been sterilized at the time when she was interviewed. Therefore, much of her contribution reflects her feelings, experiences and anger as she continued making applications and attending medical interviews which resulted in refusal. Emma had 'always known' that she did not want children of her own. She lived with a constant fear of becoming pregnant (even, she says, when she knew that it was impossible for her to be so) and had first applied for sterilization at the age of 16, and then again at 18, just before becoming pregnant and going through the stressful ordeal of abortion. The meetings with consultants were all in varying ways vexing and humiliating. She speaks of having been treated 'like a child' and feeling that she was being 'infantized' and, in many ways and at many points, her ongoing story is about her perceptions of the prejudices directed towards her as a single, child-free woman and what she describes as the power and control wielded over her by a disapproving medical profession. The following set of writing is in chronological order leading from the experience of her traumatic abortion on to a period of calm and quiet reflection. Following the exhausting, stormy and ultimately frustrating struggle of several refused applications, Emma was sterilized in June 1997.

Suffer, little children

Two rows of beds, like cattle herded in and out on the same day. The four of us in a row facing the women on the other side, facing their D&Cs as they faced ours. But ours were spelt differently – TOP. The last hurdle of the longest two weeks of my entire life. I felt like I'd been pregnant forever and I wanted myself back. I took the accusing looks in my stride. I'd expected the labour ward – where we would have been save for cuts in beds.

Pain I hadn't expected. We lay there, me and my foetus, in labour – too long, they'd left us too long. The 'mother-already' started to cry. Fear. Still. We lay in silence. Blood seeped out and through the cotton fibres like ink on paper, and the pain tiptoed then tumbled out and through my body, ripping the cells, trying to expel the alien whose pain I felt scream through me.

We lay in silence. I hadn't expected this. Don't speak. They might have changed their minds. Hide the mess. Don't make trouble. We've wasted enough of their time already. Stifled tears, hidden pain, pan-faced, don't let it out, not yet, it's not over yet. Pain, make it physical, don't scream, there's too much to come out, you won't be able to stop.

Control. They gave us injections to stop the labour pains. Emergency in theatre, we had to wait. Life before death. (They left the curtains slightly drawn, cut off from each other, my guilt-laden soulmates. Holding back the pain, the tears, the thoughts – alone.) Things started to move.

D&Cs first, leave the murderers until last. Then there were four. Me and another. The porter walked in and read out her name. She smiled at me. I was alone. The pain got worse and the blood and the tears seeped out. I mopped the tears with the sheet, I controlled my breathing – but they wouldn't stop. I was sobbing ready to explode, running around inside my head, trying to hide. Quiet. I didn't want to make a fuss. The porter came back for me. Not long. 'Do you know why you're here . . . ?' (I looked through tears into her face and tried to think through the swamp of my brain: it could be a trick question. Careful.) 'Yes.' (She had hold of my hand, I pulled away and put it back on my stomach. She probably thought I was sad because I was losing my baby. It fucking hurt.)

A younger woman emerged, nun-like in a surgical dress. She put her hand on top of mine, she stroked my head. She smiled, and I just gazed at her smile as we pressed harder and harder, pushing it down, the pain, the foetus, life, harder until my hand went numb. I didn't feel the needle. I sighed and relaxed as the drug pumped up my arm, into my body, through the pain . . .

Piece of meat, cold floor, naked, vulnerable. They tossed me onto the table, laughing, talking, what they had watched on television the night before. Opening my legs and sucking everything out. Killing. Laughing. I was unconscious yet still responsible. It was my choice. My name, my signature, on the endless pieces of paper.

I heard the noise first. Screaming. And then I felt it coming out. My voice screaming, sobbing, I let it out. My heart, brain and body bled as I let it out. Like a radiator, bleeding. 'Shut up, you're embarrassing yourself.' I screamed louder. I could make a noise. They couldn't put everything back in; they couldn't stop me doing it now; it was too late, I wanted to scream, you bastards. The religious doctor couldn't oppose my abortion on moral grounds now. I shouted words which didn't make sense to them or me. I screamed at the world which could never let me bring a child into it. I had protected my child. I was a good mother. I had killed it before they had a chance to destroy it, slowly.

'I need to go to the toilet.' I sat up, crawling on the bed. Only two nurses, and four young women, trying to pick themselves up. It was too late. I had pissed myself blood-red. They changed the sheets as I sat on the bed and I bled on the new ones. I went to the waiting room, to the others, and our guests, who wore faces of horror and disbelief.

Death, with smiles, and we were all lighting cigarettes. Tear-stained faces. Blood-stained hands. Smiling. Smoking. Throwing up. Sent back to bed. A sense of relief cut through the pain which hung about the ward. Our ward. Four human beings again, pretending to our patient visitors that nothing real or significant had happened. Their faces were white but, they said, mine looked worse. I was talking; fast, high, relieved. Telling, explaining. They loved me – didn't they? They understood? I felt so great it was over. I knew I would feel guilty forever. People would make me guilty with their unspoken opinions. But they couldn't put it back in – and they couldn't stop me from screaming now. (1993)

My scary chance of freedom

After my two counselling sessions, and after identifying my unresolved feelings of guilt from my abortion, I cried for my dead baby and I cried for my guilt and I buried them both. At 22 years of age I was again laughed out of the doctor's surgery. I had asked about sterilization: they were more interested in my cholesterol level. They won't tamper with my god-given gift.

I've had enough, this scenario could go on forever, and it isn't necessarily only because I'm 22 or only because I'm childless (like being childless is some unnatural state to be in and the only way to remove that barrier is to have a child, which defeats the whole point). I find out about my other options. To go private with Marie Stopes is £275, plus £45 for one hour of counselling. Fine!

Oh, but depending (again) on how many children I have and depending (again!) on my age.

She laughed. It wasn't a patronizing laugh – I'll give her that – but it was a laugh of reality. She didn't know how important this is to me: she wouldn't laugh at a woman with seven children – why laugh at me? Shortly afterwards, registered at a new doctors and re-prepared arguments at the ready, I steeled myself to go again through the humiliation of being viewed with suspicion as some form of psychological head case.

I met a woman who changed my life. Very calmly she gave me a leaflet on sterilization. I must make another appointment after reading it. At that meeting I spoke and she responded: eventually, she agreed to refer me.

For the first time in my life . . . you didn't dismiss me, you didn't patronize me, you didn't give me false hope. Do you know how wonderful, how beautiful that was?

Since I was nine I knew the world was shit, and knew I had sexual desire, and felt that guilt, all mixed up.

Since I was 16 I have known I don't want children.

Now, at 22 and childless, I am told that even if I pay I will have to 'prove' myself. I have no doubt. I have questioned my feelings and logic for so long.

Yet, do I have to prove myself to have a child? No! I have to fight to assert my desire and to free my body from the guilt of that desire. Your guilt, not mine. If I could abort without your baggage I could be free now, but your assumptions about my worth as a 'woman' label as wrong my sex, desire and freedom. If it wasn't wrong, would I have to fight? If I did change my mind would it affect anybody but me? So, what is the problem? It doesn't feel wrong. It feels like a chance at freedom. Is that what scares you . . . (October 1995)

Stealing the essence of me

I've always known that I didn't want children. I've never had a maternal instinct in my life and the thought of having one scares me to death. I am bitter that I have to prove myself – as if not wanting children is odd. If I don't want children, I shouldn't have sex; the answer to my desire to remain childless. Simply deny my sexual feelings, deny my desire and sexuality, and everything will be fine. A very simple logic.

I have this nightmare where I'm numb, asleep within a dream. I meet a man, usually someone famous, have great sex and then find out that I'm pregnant. Obviously I have to get married and nine months later I give birth to a baby which I've nurtured within me. That's when I wake up within the dream and the numbness subsides to reveal horror within myself. The real me emerges to the disgust of the nurses and those around me and I try to explain that this is not my baby, that I don't want it. I explain how I don't believe in marriage or motherhood as a religious or state institution which oppresses women and perpetuates the capitalist, patriarchal society.

Then I wake up: shaking, dripping with sweat, angry, sad and confused. For hours I will try to analyse this recurring dream. My conclusion is that I am scared that someone will steal my essence, the real me, my soul and conscience and I will turn into that 'something' within myself that I am fundamentally opposed to – a wife and mother. (October 1995)

Consultation . . . ? Not!

What a waste of fucking time. He had the response all worked out and didn't even ask me how I felt. The 'statistics' show that it is not advisable to sterilize me as 'we' change our minds . . . and 'although he realizes I'm an individual . . .' Well, no – he didn't realize I'm an individual because he didn't ask me any questions, just made assumptions about my body and my reasons, lumped me in with the other young women who are just as adamant as I am. But I was so angry, so fucking angry that he has the power to sit in judgement over me, make decisions on my behalf. He didn't want to hear the same reasons he'd heard before from some pathetic little girl who would inevitably change her mind – that's if he even 'allowed' me the luxury of having a mind.

He would never have to fear pregnancy, never have to check every five minutes for the bleeding which would quell the panic attacks which make me believe I'm pregnant. He wasn't fucking interested, and when I suggested that he could have sent a letter with his worked-out refusal, and that this meeting was a waste of time, he used it to imply that I wasn't really serious! I might have wasted my own time but not his! – and he apologized in the face of the statistics, and apologized for being patronizing, yet was patronizing, anyway . . . (November 1995)

Beyond your intellect – above your reason

I haven't written anything for a while. The space I had, to contemplate all the reasons why I don't want children, seems unimportant when faced with the reality of a system which seeks to silence me. I used to write poetry and prose, moving with my feelings to extract the reasoned logic surrounded by the essence of me. Now I construct academic essays and conference papers in my head because you made me cry out of frustration and anger. If you make someone into a child through your behaviour then they behave like one.

I don't see the end any more, just a drudge through contradictions you don't see. You don't observe how referring to my 'failed long-term relationship' shows how you deny my individuality and subjectivity. You don't see that you deny me the right to make decisions about my own body, you don't observe, or you don't care. You don't see yourself doing anything but serving your own interests and mine. Watching your back and my womb.

You take away my choice to choose by giving me an option I don't want. I don't want that choice. I want to deny that possibility of something I don't wish to experience. I want to control my body to the point where you no longer do.

But these arguments are futile, so I try to see the construction of academic logic which goes beyond your intellect, which places me above you in reason, but not in my body, not in reality. So we play a game of money, class, gender and power – but I have none.

However many fancy theories or rationalities I can produce to argue my case, you have the power to dismiss and refuse me and you so readily do that. You do not listen, you don't want to listen because it doesn't fit what you perceive me to be. So I feel this frustration and anger, which I must silence to play our sordid game, but this shouldn't be a game, this is important and if you had any respect for me as a person, you would see that. (January 1996)

Waiting for clearance

I expect them to dismiss me – but I won't give up. I want to feel what my body is like without those pills. So, here I am, waiting for my consultation with the man who holds the purse and my future. I have my clothes ready to role play the young, intelligent, professional woman who knows her own mind and her own stuff. I have my arguments: financial, political, hedonistic, altruistic, medical . . . and it is up to them, now. I've put hormones into my body for the last seven years – and, no, I don't consider Norplant to be a viable alternative to sterilization. I got pregnant on such 'foolproof' ingenuity and now carry guilt as a consequence. I want to await my monthly bleeding knowing that it will arrive without the nightmares and panic attacks making me believe I'm pregnant – even when I haven't even had sex! I just want somebody to agree with me, and to legitimize what I already know – but sometimes doubt – that it is OK to have sex and desire even when you know that you don't want children. (October 1996)

Wasted time and futile arguments

It was obvious from the start that you had no intention whatsoever of considering me for sterilization – you used statistics to point out that there was a high risk that I would 'change my mind' . . . but, you didn't ask me about, or give me the opportunity to discuss with you, my individual feelings and beliefs on the subject. Yet again a member of the medical profession dismissed my concerns and beliefs without even listening to what I had to say.

You may recall that I was very upset when I left the consultation. This was because it was quite apparent that it was futile to argue with someone who had already made a life decision about my body, before even meeting with me.

Unlike you, I have spent seven years of my life taking oral contraceptive pills and subjecting my body to the hormones they contain. Unlike you, I have been through the experiences of a termination of pregnancy which was caused by the failure of the contraceptive methods that I was using to prevent pregnancy. Unlike you, I have experienced irrational panic attacks, even when for me to be pregnant is an impossibility.

The information, the refusal could more easily have been given and less time wasted, outside of a consultation. You didn't even want to know why I – an individual woman who does know her own mind – would want to be sterilized. (November 1996: from a letter to a consultant: this version unsent, later revised)

Where am I now . . .?

I'm at a place where I play a cat-and-mouse game with my GP. Every time I go to renew my prescription for the contraceptive pill – which I am sure dulls my senses and makes me ill – I propose alternative contraceptive methods. I start with sterilization: he smiles – we're both bored with this game.

I hear his usual response to which I have to agree. No, I don't want to sit and face another arrogant gynaecologist who thinks he knows more about my choices and risk than I do. 'Coil . . .?' – 'Persona . . .?'. The consultation ends up with a prescription for another six months' pills and yet another blow to my rights, as a human being, to control – in this technological age – my ability to reproduce.

It makes me angry, but I think that we both know it's a game. He certainly can't accuse me of being impatient or hysterical about it, but he knows how frustrated I am. I'm sure by the look on his face when I walk in that it frustrates him too – but not enough to do anything about it! I understand – theoretically – why they won't sterilize me. I'm a woman who lives in a society which still can't accept the eternal spinster, especially one (hetero)sexually active.

So, two years later, this is where I am. Waiting eagerly to be able to take this book to my GP when it is published and to defy him to continue the charade when faced with the TRUTH of so many women who wanted to be sterilized without having had children, and who HAVEN'T regretted their decision despite being told so many times, by doctors and consultants, that they will.

I have been encouraged so much by learning about the experiences of other women. This has given me hope and enabled me to stay calm despite a type of medical 'logic' which defies explanation within the grounded universe! I know now that making me feel stupid is intended to undermine a decision which causes 'them' so many problems. I also know that I am not alone, evil, selfish, unnatural or uncaring for wanting to do this. (April 1997)

Forward thinking

I look at the world and I don't like what I see. I live in a world where profit and power are more important than humanity and nature. I guess that if I look to how I would like to see the future, it's not about me being sterilized at all.

I want to live in a place where I could bring children into the world and where the thought of doing so wouldn't fill me with guilt and pain.

I want to live in a society which doesn't segregate and discriminate on the basis of gender, race, religion, sexuality, disability, money, power, status and technology.

I want to live in a culture where differences and individual skills are acknowledged for the contributions they make.

I want to live in a country which doesn't have to murder people in the name of borders.

I want to live in a world which takes collective responsibility for its children.

I want every child born to be cared for and respected; not abused, neglected and worse through the 'natural right' of the parent.

I often think about Margaret Attwood's *Handmaid's Tale*. I wonder how many of us it would take to change anything? I wonder how long it would take before rape and forced artificial insemination replace choice? ... and the future? I'm with Marge Piercy on that one. So, how do I see it?

I see the future in relation to the science fiction around me in today's popular 'feminist' culture. I see the future as a place where we must make choices about what we want for ourselves and our children – and I don't consider that sterilization would absolve me from that responsibility. So – if I were to be sterilized ...

... sterilization ensures that I can contribute to society in different ways without the burden of guilt that I know that I would experience and would have to endure if, indeed, I had a child. Sterilization means that I am 'free' from a biological constraint, a limit on my personal ability to fulfil my real potential as a human being.

Sterilization allows me to be sexual. The alternative is celibacy or, at least, celibacy from heterosexual activity. Maybe wanting sexual freedom and biological freedom is selfish. This is the word I hear used against people like me, but in the science fiction of reality we can put men on the moon, launch satellites, probe the universe and find life on Mars.

I don't want heaven and earth. I just want the earth in a form which rests easy on my collective social conscience. (May 1997)

... carefully, in detail, in cool phrases, Flora explained exactly to Meriam how to forestall the disastrous effect of too much sukebind and too many long summer evenings upon the female system.

Meriam listened, with eyes widening and widening.

''Tes wickedness! 'Tes flying in the face of Nature!' she burst out fearfully at last.

'Nonsense!' said Flora. 'Nature is all very well in her place, but she must not be allowed to make things untidy . . .'

(Stella Gibbons, *Cold Comfort Farm*, 1932)

You cannot choose when to have children – you can only choose when not to have them. (Margaret Leroy, 1988)

The reaction from the world is, 'hasn't got children? Weird!' (Judith, 1996)

Introduction

Background to the book

The sudden surge of media interest, early in 1995, in reports of a growing incidence of childlessness (Condy, 1995; McAllister, 1998) and an inevitable follow-up of media reports, interviews and chat shows, with their discussions and debates about such a possibility, was sufficient encouragement for speculation and warnings about the dire consequences for Britain of a decreasing population, providing also the platform for concerned comment about 'unnatural' women. It was a predictable nine-day wonder and, with media interest fading, the subject dropped from having a high profile to making occasional appearances in magazines and publications for women. Although the press gave only a brief period of time to the Family Policy Studies project and Fiona McAllister's forthcoming report, and seldom ventured beyond the 'soundbite' headline, more questions were raised about the issue than were satisfactorily answered. Not for the first time I began to consider why and how an increasing number of women appear to be rejecting motherhood as a role and avoiding mothering as an experience.

At the end of my teacher-training course in the mid-1970s, my dissertation topic (with the lengthy and rather pompous title, 'Decision-making Factors Relating to Childfree and Non-contracted Marriages') focused on what was then a relatively new trend. Doctors were willing to prescribe the contraceptive pill and women were responding to changing perceptions of heterosexual enjoyment for women as well as men. The potential for controlling personal fertility was part of newly developing awareness for the individual, slowly eroding the often lifelong distress and unhappiness of 'having to get married' as well as the shame attached to being an unmarried mother with a child who, in law and in the eyes of society, effectively had no father.

My study was in the early part of the 1970s (at the tail-end of the so-called 'sexual revolution') and I was exploring traditional and changing sexual attitudes and behaviour. My thinking around the related areas of the topic was influenced by a number of key academic books, particularly the works of Simone de Beauvoir, Shulamith Firestone and Sheila Row-botham, and the conclusion that I reached was that increased knowledge about contraception created the possibility for couples to live together prior to marrying and to postpone family life until, it seemed, the joint decision to have a child prompted the decision to wed. Some couples appeared happy to remain unwed and without having children, but I noticed also that a small number of women were writing about making personal decisions regarding their responses to motherhood and their commitment to childfree lifestyles. I had also read Ellen Peck's book *The Baby Trap* (1973) and this polemic piece of writing from one woman's highly personal viewpoint presented a robust exploration of a childfree lifestyle. Peppered with generalized references to childfree friends, conversations held with other childfree couples and scathing references to the negative aspects of parenting, I found it refreshing, stimulating and thought-provoking.

Much later, after six years of teaching and – by then – fifteen years of motherhood, I read Stephanie Dowrick and Sybil Grundberg's book, *Why Children?* (1980) and found this collection of contributions to be measured and considered in tone, with eighteen women exploring their motivations for parenting or for remaining without children. I was immensely impressed by these examples of the woman's voice: reflective and, by turn, sober, joyful, grave, rapturous, painful, serene, about the intensely female experiences of pregnancy and giving birth, the tender bonding and fiercely passionate mother–child love. Only six of the women were decidedly childfree and of these only one had been sterilized in order to ensure that she remained so. I was equally impressed by their reflections on decisions which had had such far-reaching effects on their lives and the care and thought given to the finality and possible burden of this choice. That experience, of recognizing and giving attention to the woman's voice,

2

profoundly influenced my developing feminist consciousness, providing me with a constant reference point throughout my adult life.

My initial motivations for undertaking this study are personal and, in part, the book reflects my own experiences of seeking sterilization. In 1979 I knew that I had completed my family (my two 'boys' are both now in their thirties) and wanted no more children. At the age of 32 I chose to be sterilized. My second request to be considered for sterilization was successful and dealt with swiftly by an NHS hospital in the Midlands which specialized in treating women, and took no more than three weeks from meeting the consultant to undergoing the operation. The first application, however, provided me with an experience of being patronized and summarily dealt with in ways which I found both harrowing and infuriating.

My GP was sympathetic to the reasons for my application and his referral resulted in an NHS hospital appointment. I emerged from that consultation feeling insulted and powerless, having been told that I was 'much too young and attractive' to be considered for sterilization and that there might be 'a handsome chap on a white charger' just waiting to marry me and wanting me to have his babies. The recommendation to my GP would be for me 'to return to the pill, and a letter would be written to that effect'.[1] When I reminded the consultant that I had told him that a major reason for ceasing the Pill was because of physical symptoms, including headaches and weight gain, my concern was breezily dismissed with the comment, 'Pure vanity, my dear'. Before the anger set in, I felt foolish and childlike, as though I had made an obviously ridiculous request.

At the outset of this study, and at a distance of some fifteen years, it did not occur to me that I would be hearing stories which not only were not very much different from that past experience but also, because the women in the study had had no children, in some instances were infinitely worse. Only when I began to read contemporary studies on childfree women and began to interview childfree women did I fully appreciate the deeply entrenched and controlling nature of some aspects of the medical profession. In the diary accounts about their personal experiences I read that my correspondents found that, despite presenting what they believed to be their considered choice and a logical case for sterilization – reasons identified again and again as dissatisfaction with their method of contraception – they were being judged by doctors as not capable of taking such a momentous decision for themselves. Pauline's anger spilled over into sarcasm as she told me about her applications.

> I applied to my male GP for sterilization when I was approx-
> imately 27 and was turned down because I was 'too young and
> might find another husband who wanted children', the inference
> being first, that I would want to find another husband and if my
> husband wanted children I would either have no personal choice
> and give myself over to the wisdom of a superior being, or second,
> I would become so besotted (in a fit of temporary insanity!) that I
> would succumb to the call of motherhood. I applied again at age
> 30 to another male GP and was told pretty much the same thing.
> Not surprisingly I felt powerless and angry with both of the GPs
> . . . and I have just discovered that I didn't realize just how angry
> I was until typing the last paragraph. (Pauline, aged 44).

News features on reproductive choice generally present women as acting on a whim, possibly so that they are able to pursue a career, commenting with amazement that they seem determined to resist their destiny yet, far from being a simple decision for women, confronting this 'so-called need to mother' (Hanmer, 1993) is one of the more compli-cated aspects of a woman's life. There are many sympathetically handled reports and studies which focus on the distress caused by involuntary childlessness and the medical help and treatment available: if mentioned at all, voluntarily childfree women are briefly dealt with and their voice is absent from the text. Over the past two decades and with a number of studies available, it seems that there is a developing research interest in voluntarily childfree women yet, even when they were included in the studies, the voice of electively sterilized childfree women remained uni-dentified and their significant difference was overlooked. A further omission of their voice is in the medical research field and I found that I was reading what the medical profession was saying about these women rather than hearing them tell their individual stories.

Women have absorbing and thought-provoking stories to tell about being without children in a world where this is considered not only aberrant but also an issue of social concern. Those who are frank and open about their choice will find themselves the target of curious, or more often critical, comment and, from the outset of the research, I knew that

I wanted to hear more than just a catalogue of the reasons that women give for remaining childfree and to discover how some women decide to act on their childfree choice by opting for voluntary sterilization. From my preliminary reading, I felt that I could detect a significant difference between sterilized women and women who continued using other methods of contraception and so I began to explore the differences in attitudes of the majority of childfree women in continuing with contraception over their fertile life cycle and the action of a minority of childfree women in giving up monthly contraception and opting to be sterilized.

There are a number of books based on interviews with British and American childfree women, usually married and aged in their forties-through-seventies (Dowrick and Grundberg, 1980; Veevers, 1980; Campbell, 1985; Marshall, 1993; Bartlett, 1994; Morell, 1994). I undertook a fresh review of relevant literature and research papers, also searching the various Internet websites for contributions and conversations posted on the few, mainly American, 'childfree' lists. From my list of older books, I returned to Stephanie Dowrick and Sybil Grundberg's *Why Children?*, which became the starting point for hearing the voice of individual women who had wrestled with the idea of motherhood and had reached a decision which was right for themselves and their lifestyle; and I also found that Ellen Peck's amusing and acerbic *The Baby Trap: An Outspoken Attack on the Motherhood Myth!* (1973) provided examples of the type of responses which the childfree learn to use when, in their own terms, they are under attack. For example, the answer to the remark that there will not be anyone available to take care of childfree people in their old age is briskly refuted as nonsense; 'we shall be happy and active and have many friends of all ages, as we do now – quite unlike many lonely parents who spend their days complaining about children who do not write or visit . . . '. The rather more pointed remark regarding how childfree people must be suppressing their desire for children by keeping animals is also neatly turned around on the questioner, 'no, you have a sublimated desire for dogs. You, after all, have children'.

Even when remaining good-natured, and wit and repartee aside, Ellen Peck recognized that the sober side of this type of incomprehension needed to be confronted and dealt with, particularly when responding to relatives or others who are close. Nevertheless, she did not waver in her attack on what she believed to be the tyranny of children nor did she acknowledge the pull of the maternal instinct. Indeed, the tenor of the book was a direct invitation to confront the challenge that there may be benefits to choosing a childfree lifestyle.

Other significant books in this area demonstrate the various strategies and ways of coping in social contexts and interactions where children are the norm (Veevers, 1980; Bartlett, 1994; Marshall,1993). The common point of these studies is their focus on the heterosexual partnership and cooperative decision-making of the childfree venture; for example, Elaine Campbell's study (1985) of couples who do not want children. Even the most recent study by Carolyn Morell (1994), which is most sharp in drawing attention to the significance of the new nature of childfree futures, is based on interviews with women who made their decisions as part of a couple with one choice being vasectomy for the male partner.

From my reading in the early part of the study I noticed that, even when childfree sterilized women clearly identified themselves (usually by making reference to the process of deciding and writing about the difficulties that they encountered and their often fraught experiences leading up to the operation), none of the books picked out as distinct the two groups which make up the category of voluntarily childfree women. All women who assume that they are fertile and are determined to remain childfree must continue to take precautions, and most of the research conducted to date interviewed mostly older women (aged 50-plus) who had used contraception until they were safely through the menopause. However, there is also an identifiable minority who opt to be sterilized rather than continuing using contraception. I realized that there were two distinctly different 'endings' to the women's recorded stories which were dealt with in the studies as though there was only one outcome – the childfree choice. Certainly, all of the women had chosen to remain childfree but in addition to that choice some had opted to be sterilized after ceasing using contraception, thereby making chemical, barrier or other 'by-the-month' methods obsolete.

I discerned that some women's resolve went beyond decision and into action. Although I had set out to research childfree women and their motivations, I found a separate and distinct woman's voice emerging and began to hear those who had vigorously and actively pursued voluntary sterilization, often in the face of social disapproval and medical opposition. This very small area became the focus of the research. From that point I began to focus on the choice and action of childfree sterilized women and to plan for the study.

Considerations for the study: using feminist research methods

Despite many challenges from feminist researchers, male-stream research continues to dominate research activities with its expectations that women's lives and experiences must be viewed from a traditional perspective, one which continues to insist that researchers strive to be detached or neutral when engaged in the type of research which grapples with the very stuff of people's lives: this approach has been described as a 'tyranny of methodolatory', acclaimed as good scholarship and institutionalized within the male academy (Daly, 1973, in Humm, 1989). However, the well-established field of feminist research insists that the totality of the research process is of importance, including the interaction between researcher and researched (Stanley and Wise, 1983) with a relationship which is non-hierarchical, non-authoritarian and non-manipulative (Reinharz, 1983). Feminists agree that the primary purpose of under-taking feminist research is that it must have the intent of benefiting women in some way; 'it must be consciously partial, be research from below, create change by involvement in women's liberation, be consciousness raising, and be part of collective discussion with women' (Mies, 1983, in Humm, 1989).[2]

The study method for this work needed to be rigorous, qualitative in nature and based on feminist research methods, especially those that focus on patriarchy as a primary means of women's oppression.[3] So as to use the personal language and lived experiences of women participants as a major feature in presenting their individual stories of childfree lifestyles and the transition from contraception to sterilization involved me in thinking about the best strategies for organizing and collecting the information which would also provide opportunities for the women to present their choices and decisions within their life contexts. Essential, too, was making provision for the opportunity for 'conscious partiality' (Klein, 1983) which would allow me, a sterilized woman albeit having had children, to place myself within the study with the acknowledgement that my presence as a researcher affects both response and outcome. Further, I did not want to collect merely a chronology of events by choosing a research method which would allow the women participants to list their experiences yet leave no space for their emotional response. Also vital was ensuring that the research method was sufficiently flexible for women to recount the practical aspects of applying for and undergoing sterilization, whilst also having space for them to communicate their determination as powerful agents in personal decisions and actions.

I decided to use a semi-structured questionnaire which additionally invited women to write a parallel and complementary 'diary' of events, to be followed by a narrative interview – a conversation with a purpose: this format seemed to encompass the potential for maximizing how the women would present their stories (Burgess, 1995). An inflexible approach, which is so often the hallmark of structured questions, would have prevented the women from having the opportunity for the required freedom of expression (Hunt and Symonds, 1995). I intended to build pictures about the women's life experiences from their responses to a questionnaire, and take extracts from written diaries and interviews, wherever possible using their own words.

More formally structured interviewing, with closed questions (yes or no responses especially), was found to leave the person being interviewed feeling that they had been interrogated (Cohen and Manion, 1994), whereas the open-ended questioning of the semi-structured interview invites and encourages interviewees to respond using their own language and style of speaking. Other feminist researchers working with women use this approach and recognize that, by writing a diary, women examine social and psychological problems and can be their own theorist (Humm, 1989). Used as a feminist and psychological tool, interviewing facilitates an understanding of the ways in which women evaluate their lives and experiences (Phoenix, in Burman, 1990), thus the very act of writing can be political for women and women's power is extended through organizing thoughts on paper, expressing feelings and responding to others (Chester and Nielsen, 1987).

My opening to the questionnaire focused on the basic details and personal profile of the women themselves. Beyond that, my initial intention was to extend the study area further than only married women or women in heterosexual relationships, as other books focus on joint decision-making by couples (usually married). I wanted to discover whether the sterilized women who responded to my invitation to talk about their experiences were making choices and reaching their own childfree decisions regardless of the opinions or influences of a male partner and so one of the questions asked women about this part of the process in reaching their decision.

I was very wary of making any assumption about a woman's sexual identity being a reason for her deciding not to have children and so the questionnaire asked women how they would describe their sexuality. I began the research with an assumption that women who identify as heterosexual may choose to remain childfree, that bisexual women and women who identify as lesbians can and do make the choice to become mothers and that the reasons for making any choice relating to motherhood would be broadly similar for all women regardless of their sexuality.

I wanted to ensure that women's self-identified disabilities were represented and so the questionnaire asked women to say whether they were challenged in some way or had a disabling condition. Women were asked to identify any pressures on them to be sterilized because of their conditions as a way of highlighting any medical decisions which smacked of eugenics, a position often invoked to justify controlling the reproductive rights and potential of women who are not considered suitable to have children.

Previous studies of childfree women show an age range from women in their forties through to seventies. I wanted as full an age range as possible to be represented and the ages of women in this study range from 22 to 51 when first contacted. This was important to my tentative suggestion of difference in the choices made between women who remain childfree whilst continuing to use contraceptives up to and through menopause, and women who cease using contraceptives and opt for sterilization when young.

There are few studies which question a commonly held assumption that, because white Europeans and Americans form the basis for most research and of books about childfree women, it is only white women who make such a choice. Although Carolyn Morell (1994) identifies a number of American works which belie that assumption, ultimately her study also fits that characterization. I gave much thought as to how to reach women who could speak and write about their experiences from the richly diverse cultural and religious contexts which exist in contemporary Britain. This wish was not realized and all of the women who initially responded and those who became participants are white and British. Each one of the stories is valuable and absorbing but, regrettably, the study does not have any perspective other than from the UK white majority culture.

Dealing with fertility and reproduction is an issue for all women of every class which, in Britain, is seen as a vital research consideration. I acknowledge that class issues may be identified in this study but allow the childfree women's own words to describe their lives, undertakings and activities, their work and leisure time, rather than using scales or even terms such as working class or middle class. Educational background and achievement, economic status and women's knowledge and choice of contraception and birth control may all have a bearing on the personal choice of methods and strategies used to control fertility, but the diversity of the women's backgrounds (not just their current status) made me cautious about the class dimensions of such a small study group. The range of present and past lifestyles and occupations covers women unwaged and working in the voluntary sector, on the factory floor, in public services such as social work, education and counselling and psychology, as well as the Inland Revenue, medicine, law and the Church. The private sector and private enterprise are also represented, although probably the most unusual past job was Jude's – she was a shepherd.

The voice of childfree women: using diaries and interviews to tell women's stories

Most of the women who wrote the diary accounts of their experiences had never before put pen to paper as a way of recording their thoughts and innermost feelings. Although some had written to GPs or consultants whilst waiting for decisions to be made about their applications for sterilization, responding to my advertisement and then talking and writing to me was the first time most of the women had further explored their choice to remain childfree and their decision to be sterilized. Their initial letters ranged from one to several pages, typed or handwritten, inviting me to be in touch and giving me a glimpse of the women behind the stories. Every story was absorbing, with numerous similarities between them, and a number were full of anger and pain at not being taken seriously, being ignored and refused, whilst also showing a strength and determination to keep on trying even in the face of rejection. Two written accounts in particular stood out for me as going beyond the personal considerations essential for maintaining the determination to continue, presenting emotional details and political insights which underpinned and further established the validity of the women's struggle.

Emma was one of the first respondents and is a women who knew from the age of 16 that she never wanted children. Her detailed writing documents the painful journey from deciding on sterilization to achieving her goal ('Emma's Story' provides extracts from her personal diary). She feels that she was forced to fight her way to being taken seriously and so, despite having to confront disapproval, refusal and medical intransigence, her reflections demonstrate the many and diverse ways in which women's independence and maturity is compromised. Her voice is significant in the study because, at the time of her response to the advertisement, she was in the process of making applications and being turned down; experiences which, in varying degrees, she found stressful and humiliating. In this way she charted an ongoing and similar journey to the experiences of the other women who all write in retrospect. At the age of 23 Emma fell into the category 'young woman without children' which every service – even Marie Stopes – is cautious about considering for sterilization. Emma had experienced the trauma of an unwanted pregnancy and the physical and emotional pain of abortion and, at the beginning of our correspondence, she had almost given up on being considered for sterilization but was awaiting two decisions; one from a consultant at an NHS hospital and one from a registered charity for which she was saving money in case she was successful. In April 1997 a Marie Stopes clinic referred Emma for sterilization despite, in their words, 'not agreeing' with her reasons. In the time it took for her to be considered, the cost had risen considerably but she was delighted and relieved to feel in control of her own fertility and to know for certain that she will remain childfree.

Jude's diary was fifteen pages of closely written script covering events and situations, emotions, rages, anger, actions and reactions, and many reflections. On first receiving it I found that I was reading at an increasing pace, rushing through the story towards its conclusion, feeling that I could sense the urgency with which she wrote, more and more furiously, her story spilling out onto the pages, her thoughts and writing jumping between describing the process in a practical way and then offering deeply emotional disclosures. Jude's diary, the follow-up interview in which she spoke about the process of writing, and then her reflections on the interview and what it meant for her, confirmed how essential it is to approach the task of interviewing with caution and sensitivity, asking questions and listening to women as they tell their stories, and as they compose their own inner realities through personal narrative (Jude's 'Reflections on a Process' concludes Chapter 5). From the outset I wanted to provide an opportunity for each woman to tell her story in reflective, diary form and through interviews, so that each would construct her own deeply personal, written and oral history, thus allowing sufficient space for the woman's voice to be heard.

The early stage of the fieldwork was to advertise for contacts from 'voluntarily childfree sterilized women' using *Everywoman*, a monthly women's magazine (now defunct), and *Counselling*, the journal of the British Association for Counselling. Similar advertisement 'flyers' were sent to a cluster of local GP practices, to local NHS and private hospitals and to a number of charity-funded organizations and clinics which provide information, advice and practical support and help on fertility, contraceptive and abortion issues; in particular, Marie Stopes and family planning clinics and community healthcare services. The 38 letters received in the first two months were as a result of the crucial word 'childfree' being omitted from the advertisement in *Everywoman*: thirteen women responded who had been sterilized after completing their family and they were thanked but not included in the study. I attempted to use the 'snowball' method to provide some of my study group but I soon discovered that most childfree sterilized women do not know anyone else like themselves: only two women were contacted through word-of-mouth, being friend-of-a-friend. Of a remaining group of 25, two chose not to continue, leaving a final self-selected study group of 23 voluntarily childfree sterilized women.

The women respondents used what I had developed as a 'prompt-style' questionnaire, encouraging them to write a 'diary' in their own discursive style but also answering 57 questions clustered under nine headings. A letter accompanying the questionnaire asked them to include details which would throw further light on their responses. They were encouraged to reflect upon their memories about early life experiences, especially if they were able to identify personal reasons for later reproductive decisions; to provide details of early and adult sexual activity with or without contraceptive precautions; to record the practical and emotional details of the process leading up to the sterilization operation; and to comment on their lives immediately after the operation and since. The focus was on a variety of features which I had identified from my background reading on childfree women and the issues which had been highlighted by them in previous research: how did they know that they did not want children?; had they gone through a process of choosing not to have them?; what contraceptive methods had they used and what was the outcome of any pregnancy scares?; what was their initial motivation for considering sterilization and how did they go about finding out how to apply?; did they tell anyone and, if so, how did other people react to the news?; if they were in a partnership did the partner have any say in the decision?; in both practical and emotional terms did they find it easy to move from decision to action?; how did they recall the medical procedure? Finally, were there any regrets?

The style of questionnaire was useful in establishing many similarities in the women's accounts and the ways in which their various journeys towards sterilization are comparable and the flexibility of the questionnaire was shown in its open invitation to add to or extend its scope as seemed appropriate with separate diary narratives allowing each woman's individuality and personality to emerge: the follow-up interviews then built on that foundation. This approach highlighted and effectively documented the similarities between the individual women's unique stories and illustrated their determination – their active agency – in seeking and undergoing sterilization.

Examining and exploring the rich material of the written diaries would assist in charting the women's life decisions and also give information about their considerations in choosing to be sterilized rather than continuing with other forms of contraception. I also contacted and interviewed a number of GPs, doctors and specialists in family planning centres and clinics, and consultant gynaecologists and obstetricians working within the NHS and in private practice. Several other specialist consultants also took the time to answer my written or telephone enquiries and managers and directors working in clinics in the charity and voluntary sectors were immensely helpful and supportive, showing a keen interest in the study and being a source of much additional valuable insight and information. It was possible and practical for me to minimize travelling time by meeting women in close proximity to each other. The ordinary pressures of work and other commitments meant that I could not arrange to meet five of the women: they were so far from any of my planned round trips that, for a one-hour interview, I would have spent many hours travelling several hundreds of miles. These interviews were conducted by phone, further letters and occasionally via e-mail.

I found the interviews with the diarists to be stimulating, inspiring, often amusing and full of details of each woman's progress from how they first decided that sterilization would be the most efficient and effective contraception for them, on to taking action and realizing that decision. Some of the diaries and interviews also described anger, frustration and feelings of helplessness in the face of what they described as blatant insensitivity, meted out to them by a medical profession seemingly intent on disempowering and infantizing them.

Each interview opened with an informal discussion with the woman about the scope of the study. I made a short statement about the feminist perspective which underpins my work, indicating that I wanted the interview to be as relaxed as possible and hoping that we could engage in a dialogue. I introduced my intention of using a tape recorder so as to eliminate the need for lengthy and obtrusive note-taking and asked each woman for permission to do so: all agreed and I further explained that I would either return or destroy the tapes once the study was published. I intended to listen to the story, choosing appropriate times to check details or ask for clarification in order not to break the flow. I also invited the woman to ask me questions which had arisen either about my motivations and intentions for the study, or where she needed to clarify how I would deal with her personal contribution to the book. Ann Oakley's work on interviewing women had impressed me (Oakley, 1974, and in Roberts, 1981) and I wanted to ensure that the women did not perceive me as being an interrogator asking all the questions and remaining aloof (or detached, or neutral) from the 'stuff' of the interview. It was important for me to know that I was not oppressive nor inappropriately intrusive and so I stated that I would try to be aware of any signalled boundaries but that I welcomed being told if my questions strayed over limits: this principle, reciprocally, also applied to me. Most questions were functional and it seemed that my reassurance, and invitation to be questioned as well as doing the questioning, contributed to the generally relaxed atmosphere of each interview.

As an opener to each interview, and to make my personal agenda for the meeting reasonably clear, I indicated which parts of their written story had especially interested me and asked for a more detailed verbal account. All of the women responded with openness and a number of them commented that it was the first time that they had spoken in depth about their experience. After each interview I listened to the tape and compared spoken details with the written diary. I was searching for those features of each story which provided similarities with the experiences of other women – and there were many – as well as the significant features which made each story highly individual. Each tape was partially transcribed for identified significant sections. I wanted the women themselves to emerge as central figures in the book, and not merely appear as 'disembodied voices' within quotation marks and so I constructed short 'cameos' of each woman, drawing on the data available in her returned questionnaire and the detail of her personal diary. Once this was done, I could see that presenting the women through the medium of these profiles allowed them to be more easily identified, and so two copies of the cameo were sent to each woman, one to keep and the other to be signed, dated and returned with any corrections, or with changes to preferred name, place or job description.

Most women returned the cameos unaltered and allowed the use of their first names, but several opted to change their name. Others asked that small but significant details were omitted or made less identifiable, for example, 'a city in the north of England' instead of the city name, or 'within the Civil Service' rather than using a job title. One woman was concerned about the 'overt homophobia which is still alive and well within the profession', and asked that certain identifying personal details were removed. Two women whom I was unable to interview felt that the cameos did not accurately reflect who they are and we acknowledged the problem which the missing personal interviews had caused. I felt that I did not have sufficiently 'rounded' views of them and so, after further phone calls and written diary additions, I completely rewrote the cameos, which they then accepted.

When the cameos were returned finally, there were also many personal cards and notes from the women giving updates on their lives and events. Several commented and reflected on how the process had affected them and most expressed anticipation for seeing the book in print. This confirmed for me the importance of providing opportunities which enable women to use their own voices to represent themselves and the detail of how they make sense of their own lives. In the following section the central place in this work of the real subjects of the book is established, with the profiles introducing and presenting the individual stories of the women. These contributions, I feel, bring to life this study of childfree women who have elected to be sterilized.

The women diarists

There are many stereotypes which supposedly identify the characteristics of childfree women: 'selfish' and 'abnormal' are among the milder descriptions. Like some other minority groups they have had a bad press yet they emerge from this study as neither better nor worse than anyone else. Women without children may be childfree but they are not all child-haters; they may have clear ideas of the pattern and goals of their future lives but they are not all selfish career women; they may come from a diversity of family backgrounds but not all are only children; they may have experienced some emotional upheaval but they are not overly disturbed or unbalanced; and few of the 23 claimed outright to be feminists. No more odd or different from members of society in general, they may not have children but they are real women, except in that they are called upon to account for their reproductive decisions in a variety of ways which are not experienced by women who are already mothers or women who seek motherhood.

Jean, from the north of England, aged 46: Jean is white, European and identifies herself as heterosexual. An only child, she was 10 years old when a sister was stillborn. She is now Anglican although she was brought up Methodist. Married at 21 and divorced at 32, she married her present husband when she was 41 and he was 68. Jean works as a staff development officer and counsellor and counsellor trainer at a university in the north of England.

Jean had planned a career in the Church. She wished to be a deaconess; at that time, they were not allowed to marry so she never considered having a family and always 'felt uncomfortable' around children. Her method of contraception before sterilization was the Pill which she began two months prior to marriage. She had one scare and had a pregnancy test which was negative. Her first request for sterilization was when she was 32 but her woman GP refused to refer her. Jean and her first husband discussed children and decided to remain childfree, then separated before sterilization was considered. She says that she would not then have entered any future relationship which compromised that decision. A counsellor, as are most of her friends, there was no formal counselling – and she did not think she would have found counselling personally useful – but she felt that there would have been support had she sought it. Jean was 36 when the NHS hospital operation was carried out and, despite

INTRODUCTION

having been turned down once, she never thought of giving up, or changing her mind. The operation itself was very straightforward and she never had any regrets. Jean has since had a hysterectomy and says that this was the best feature of all; 'no more periods!'.

Jude, from the north of England, aged 31: Jude is white, English and identifies herself as heterosexual although she is open to the possibility of change. She is the youngest of three, with two brothers, and is now atheist, although she was brought up Methodist. Jude is single, never married and has been in her monogamous relationship for eight and a half years. She has always been a feminist, is politically active and a shop steward, and is currently involved in a number of campaign-based activities. She works full-time as a crisis counsellor within the Social Services and is a part-time carer for a friend with AIDS. Her past jobs have included work on farms and she has been a shepherd.

Jude has always known that she never wanted children and has never had any maternal feelings. Her method of contraception before sterilization included safe sex, with condoms, a low-dose pill and occasional breaks using condoms or having non-penetrative sex. Jude has not had an abortion but would have done so if necessary, as she lived in constant fear of pregnancy and always used a self-test to check on frequent scares. Her partner is very supportive but Jude's decision to be sterilized was made regardless of any relationship, and she would have pursued sterilization even if single or not in a long-term relationship. Despite some internalized pressure – that perhaps she could not really trust her own feelings – she developed confidence that she wanted to remain childfree, acknowledging that children would 'massively limit' her life. As a counsellor, although she did not seek formal counselling on this issue, she believes that some form of positive discussion with other childfree women would have helped. Counselling after the operation may have helped her to deal with the response of other people, as she was aware that people could not tolerate her decision to be childfree. Sterilization ended all possibilities of motherhood and they became outraged and offended. The operation was carried out when Jude was 31 (a few months before interview) in an NHS hospital. Because of the constant fear of unwanted pregnancy, her reaction is one of total relief and liberation. She feels that sterilization was the 'only logical answer' and was a natural progression from otherwise unsatisfactory contraceptive methods.

Judith, from the north of England, aged 46: Judith is white, English, and identifies herself as 'mostly heterosexual'. She is the youngest of four, with two sisters and one brother, and describes herself as a humanist although she is not a member of any such organization. She is now single, was married at 22, divorcing after six years. By profession she is a social worker and works as a manager in the voluntary sector. Judith is a woman respondent who has given birth but, by her own definition, she considers herself to be childfree.

Judith has always been very committed to her work but, having been brought up in a conventional family, assumed that she would have children. She decided on sterilization around the time of her thirty-fifth birthday, not having met a man to whom she wanted to make a life commitment, and acknowledging that she would be unable to combine work and children single-handedly. When 17 years old and not using contraception Judith had a baby which was adopted. She was prescribed the Pill and carried on taking it more or less continuously from the age of 19, although for some months, and if she was between relationships, she stopped the Pill and did not use anything else. Her decision went beyond the purely personal and included global population concerns and issues of holocaust, poverty and violence. She had made no previous requests for sterilization nor did she receive counselling or professional advice. After considering verbal and written information, she was sterilized in an NHS hospital when 35. She prefers to look forward rather than back but admits to very occasional regrets at not having brought up a child, mainly because of the secret pregnancy and adoption of her baby when she was young. She wonders what it would be like to be proud of being pregnant rather than being left with negative memories of that experience.

Vicky, from the south-east of England, aged 42: Vicky is white, European, is a 'fairly straight' heterosexual and identifies that she suffers from asthma, eczema, labyrinthitis and overwork. She is an only child and was Christian fundamentalist but is now Quaker. Vicky is divorced and in what she describes as 'a long-term eccentric relationship'. She is an inspector of taxes.

Despite having had a traditional childhood, Vicky never seriously considered having children except during a four-month period before her ex-husband was found to have a condition which led to his sterility. Eventually her reaction to this was relief but the hospital registrar was offended when Vicky was 'not devastated' at not being able to have babies. Her present partner also expressed no desire for children, although had he done so this would not have affected her personal determination to remain childfree. Vicky's only scare coincided with a change to the mini pill. Her first tentative enquiry about sterilization was when she was 34 and she describes the GP as being rather 'self-righteous' whilst he was discussing his refusal with her. Her successful application took approximately eight months from start to finish and she was sterilized in an NHS hospital. Vicky says that the consultant refused ligation on the grounds that he would 'only clip childfree women'. She has no regrets and, after reading other books about childfree women, identifies completely with those who acknowledge their dislike of babies and children.

Jill, from London, aged 40: Jill is white, born in UK and describes herself as primarily heterosexual, although her friends say she is an 'honorary dyke'. She is the younger of two sisters and was brought up as Methodist, now having no religious beliefs or practice. She believes that she is still technically married, and now lives alone with her cat, although she is in a relationship with a man. She is a senior official for a trades union.

Jill never had any kind of maternal urge and has always known that she didn't want children, which was confirmed for her after a late-period scare. She believes that to be a parent is at least an eighteen-year, one-way commitment which she was not prepared to make. She used the Pill for six years, then endured three years with an IUD which caused her pain and heavy bleeding. Jill did not even try to obtain an NHS operation, informing rather than consulting her GP about her decision: he was extremely hostile. She was sterilized when 26 after consultation at a Marie Stopes clinic and she chose clips because she was told there were fewer menstrual problems after the operation. Jill was unhappy at continuing to rely on the Pill or IUD, she has no regrets about her sterilization and believes strongly that the NHS should make much more extensive provision for the reproductive decisions of women and men.

Sally, from London, aged 46: Sally is English, white, heterosexual and, except for her 'extreme myopia', is not disabled or challenged. She has one older sister and was brought up Protestant, becoming 'staunchly religious' in her teens and now being a 'staunch atheist'. At the time of interview, Sally was going through a divorce after ten years of marriage. She is self-employed as a freelance book-keeper and has branched out into sales.

Sally was always quite sure that she never wanted children even when she was a child herself. She has never been pregnant and found the question about 'choice' a strange one feeling that, as she did not have the slightest interest in having a child, she did not choose not to have one. At 24 she had ovarian cancer, losing one ovary and fallopian tube. Her doctors became wary about prescribing oral contraceptives because of this, but she was loath to use any other method which was less reliable than the Pill. In 1981 she was sterilized after consultations with the family planning clinic and then the British Pregnancy Advisory Service which arranged the hospital and operation. She felt no need to talk to anyone else as she was not seeking help to confirm her decision. As Sally's sex life improved dramatically after the operation, she believes that her fear of becoming pregnant may have been more deep-rooted than she realized. She says now that she has never had a single regret about the operation.

Geraldine, from Essex, aged 42: Geraldine is white, European and identifies herself as heterosexual. She describes herself as working class and agnostic, and is the eldest in a family of three children. Geraldine is twice divorced, has a background in the civil service and at the time of the interview had taken a severance package and was working as a carer. She has a master's degree and is currently studying to become a chiropodist.

Geraldine says that she always knew that she did not want children which, with hindsight, she relates to observing the control her father had over her mother. She suffered a miscarriage shortly before her eighteenth birthday and was offered the Pill whilst in hospital, continuing with this until it was felt that she should have a break after such a long time. This precipitated the decision to ask for sterilization, as the lower level of reliability and safety of the alternatives was unacceptable. There was enormous pressure from the family of her first husband, who 'were appalled' at her lack of desire to start a family. She made her own personal decision to remain childfree, although her partner did offer to have a vasectomy. She was very wary of counselling and discussed her decision only with her husband, the GP and the NHS hospital in the north-west of England where, after six months on the waiting list, the sterilization operation was carried out. Whilst counselling was not offered at any stage, Geraldine says that she would have viewed it as a method designed to stop her getting the sterilization. Unfortunately, four years after the sterilization, an ectopic pregnancy almost cost Geraldine her life: an ovarian cyst six months after that and then a total hysterectomy after a further six months, left Geraldine feeling that whilst she could not say she has no regrets she can say that she would 'still make the same decision tomorrow!'.

Linda L., from the north of England, aged 30: Linda L. is white, European, is not disabled or challenged and identifies herself as heterosexual. She is the youngest of three girls and describes herself as atheist. Widowed after only six months of marriage, to her partner of almost five years, she is now 'single but cohabiting'. Linda L. works as a personal assistant to a female independent financial adviser.

Linda L. could see how much having children drained her mother and so she says she has always known she did not want children. This feeling grew stronger and has been reinforced by her life experiences. Her main method of contraception prior to sterilization was the Pill but, after a period when she was not sexually active, she decided not to renew her prescription, for a short while relying on condoms or withdrawal. A major reason for sterilization was a reconsideration of the effect of the chemicals on her body. Linda L. was first refused sterilization in 1994 when she was 28 on the grounds of her age, with the doctor stating that she may possibly change her mind. During the two years before the operation she used a diaphragm and contraceptive jelly but was constantly aware of a higher failure rate than with the Pill. At the beginning of 1996 she had a scare which proved negative, but this confirmed her determination to be sterilized. She says that if necessary she would have considered and undergone abortion. She did not consult anybody except her GP but discussed the idea with friends, family and her partner. The operation was privately funded and carried out in a Nuffield Hospital. She is aware that being childfree is probably still considered against the norm in society but has no regrets. After the operation she experienced some discomfort and a slight loss of libido for a few weeks but, she says, 'the freedom is exhilarating!'.

Pauline, from Cheshire, aged 44: Pauline is white, European and identifies herself sexually as 'still exploring'. She is the middle child of three and describes herself as having a 'spiritual identity' but is not religious. Pauline has been married twice, the first time for three years, divorcing at 25; the second marriage lasted for five and half years and she was widowed at 38. Her current six-year relationship is with a man seventeen years younger. She is a trained secretary and personal assistant and works part-time as a freelance counsellor and trainer in stress management and assertiveness.

Pauline says that, although she cannot pinpoint when she first identified that she did not want a child, she feels that there is a link with the question of her sexual identity. She has sympathy for the idea that 'children look after you when you get old' but feels that it is a selfish motive. She remembers that she stalled her first husband's wish to have children and, in her second marriage, she had mixed feelings when she experienced an unplanned pregnancy because of the traumatic diagnosis of her husband's cancer. The pregnancy ended in a miscarriage at ten weeks. She had severe difficulties with the various contraceptive methods available including the Pill and, when relying on condoms, had a scare which led to her taking morning-after precautions and she first applied for sterilization after her divorce when she was 27 and again at the age of 30. To her extreme anger she was turned down each time because of medical opinions that she might find another husband. She discussed her decision with her mother who, because of Pauline's age, was very supportive. Her decision was made 'within the comfort' of her current long-term relationship and she was eventually sterilized in an NHS hospital when she was 40. Although she has never regretted her decision, there are times when she wonders what motherhood might have been like.

Linda R., from Cheshire, aged 48: Linda R. is white, English, heterosexual and not disabled or challenged except for symptoms of a condition known as fibromyalgia (body pains). She is the eldest of two with a younger brother and describes herself as definitely unreligious, disliking organized religion, but is 'new age', believes in reincarnation and having a 'spiritual identity'. She is separated from her husband and has recently filed for a divorce after living apart for four years. Currently, she is in a relationship but lives alone. She works full-time as a staff counsellor and welfare officer in the public sector, and was a past carer for her husband who suffers from MS.

Linda R. says that she did not plan not to have children. Married in the early 1970s, like most young married couples at that time she and her husband 'probably assumed' that they would have children. They reviewed this situation periodically but having children was not on the agenda, and definitely not after her husband's illness was diagnosed. Both sets of parents were supportive and understood the reasons why, although they were sad not to be grandparents. When their GP suggested it would probably be better not to have children, Linda R. feels that she probably 'hid behind such a convenient excuse'. Her husband offered to have a vasectomy but, because of his condition and because she was having an extramarital relationship, she felt it was necessary that it was she who should take the initiative. Before the sterilization she used the Pill for eleven years then, after telling her that she must cease using it, her GP refused to prescribe the mini-pill. She says he was 'less than helpful' in advising her on alternative methods. His suggested mechanical methods were not a real alternative for her so she did not ask him to refer her through the NHS but went straight to a Marie Stopes clinic. There was no counselling but she discussed her reasons with a male counsellor who checked for pregnancy, and told her that a D&C was part of the procedure. The operation took place in a private hospital in South Manchester. Linda R. is emphatic that she has 'never, ever regretted' the sterilization as it gave her freedom from worry, allowing her to maintain a loving and supportive extramarital relationship throughout what was an increasingly difficult marriage.

Anne T., from Derbyshire, aged 52: Anne T. is white, English, and identifies herself as heterosexual. She is an only child and an atheist. She is divorced, now single, and is an officer in an education authority.

Anne T. says that she did not want children and could not imagine children in her life. The development and continuation of her career is very important to her. She did not want a relationship that could include the possibility of having children and she experienced no conflicts in reaching the decision to remain childfree. Prior to sterilization she used the Pill but says that her starting point for finding out about sterilization was age and the dangers of continued Pill usage. She did not seek counselling and did discuss her plans with a female friend which she found very positive, although says that her parents do not know about the decision. Most of her friends do not have children although a few chose to have them. Once she had made her decision, she found that she was able to get the essential and necessary information very easily and the process, on the whole, was smooth and untroubled, her male GP making an immediate referral. She was prepared for questions about any change of mind and was able to field them successfully. The sterilization was agreed and planned to take place in an NHS hospital when the consultant diagnosed fibroids. After being admitted to hospital for a hysterectomy, an ovarian cyst was discovered and so she underwent surgery for its removal and her tubes were tied at the same time. Apart from the after-effects of the ovarian cyst operation – which were not really connected with the sterilization – Anne T. has no regrets and she found the process very simple.

Sandy, from Berkshire, aged 36: Sandy is white, 'London Irish', says that she is over the average weight for her height and suffers from mild asthma. She is married for the second time and identifies herself as heterosexual adding 'because I've never tried anything else'. She is an only child and says that she is atheist. Sandy works as a nurse, was accepted as a voluntary bereavement counsellor, and spends her spare time with a cat rescue organization.

Sandy has memories of wanting many children when she was a child herself but, after dreaming that she was pregnant when in her early twenties, remembers feeling terrified. That was when her feeling of not wanting children 'really gelled'. As a nurse, and aware of the procedure through theatre work, she thought it was not worth applying for steriliza-tion when she was younger, and she was 32 before giving any consideration to sterilization as an alternative to her various methods of contraception. She used the Pill, took occasional breaks using condoms and has not had an abortion or used the morning-after pill, but there were some pregnancy scares after unprotected sex. Her decision was a personal one regardless of future relationships, and the main reason for choosing to have the operation rather than a vasectomy for her husband was, she says, 'my body – my decision'. She did not visit a counsellor and feels it would not have helped, but did discuss the decision with husband, mother and friends and took professional advice on methods from the local family planning clinic. Her GP made an immediate referral but, although he knew Sandy, the gynaecologist would only consider her application after a further year had passed, as he believed that there are some women who ask for sterilization who do not really want it. After waiting two years, and at nearly 35, Sandy underwent sterilization in an NHS hospital and now feels happy and relieved and totally commited to her decision. Since the interview, Sandy and her husband have decided to part, and she says that she feels that her decision is even more justified, she is totally happy with what she did and is 'thoroughly enjoying the single life with five cats!'.

Heather, from Derbyshire, aged 41: Heather is white and, because she was adopted, has limited knowledge of her birth parents and background, saying that her adoptive parents are working-class 'old style conservatives' although describing herself as 'a Socialist'. She is the elder of two adopted girls, with an older step-brother, and believes that she has no (known) disabilities or challenges. She says that she has only experienced heterosexual relationships and her first marriage ended in divorce after five years. She lived with her present husband for three years before marrying him. Heather works as a student adviser in a university.

Heather was 'crazy about babies' and little children when she was young but that faded away. She never really bothered about having children and had an unplanned pregnancy and termination when 17. She remembers that a childfree woman inspired her to pursue her own goals and she began to focus on career development. Her first husband was very traditional and she was aware that she could not have both a career and a family. Before sterilization, Heather used the Pill for ten years but was disturbed by reports of associated health risks. Alternative methods were not acceptable and she began to enquire about sterilization. She would not have welcomed discussion about her decision and did not seek 'advice' on the issue. Heather's request for sterilization was at the age of 28 and because the examination revealed a large ovarian growth (a benign cyst) the operation was speedily arranged and carried out in an NHS hospital: the sterilization was then secondary and she cannot remember much about it.

Heather is the only childfree woman in this study to regret no longer being able to bear a child. Her reasons are related to her love and care for the younger son of her sister, who died aged 34. Heather and her present husband then experienced parenthood and she considered a reversal in order to attempt to have a child. After intense discussion and much consideration, which included the possibility of their not succeeding, they decided not to go ahead. They do still have the opportunity to see the child and she now deeply regrets her decision to be sterilized. (Heather's story about her regrets is included in the Appendix.)

Anne D., from Wales, aged 40: Anne D. is of Irish and English parentage although she 'feels Welsh'. She is married and describes herself as heterosexual. She was raised Church of England, now atheist, and is a self-employed artist.

Anne D. cannot remember when she first identified that she did not want children as she 'just always knew'. This caused great stress and during her school years she went to great lengths to ensure that no one found out in case they believed her to be 'a freak'. Marriage and children was the main topic of conversation and she learned early on how to play what she described as 'the game'. She realizes now how very hard it was for her as a young girl to find the courage to be so different from her peers. Prior to the sterilization she used the Pill, having occasional breaks, and there were times when she was celibate. On several occasions she did have scares, probably through late periods, which were very stressful, and times when she felt helpless and out of control. Anne D. first approached her GP for advice about sterilization when she was 27 years old. He was reluctant to refer her but she 'stuck at it' and when eventually she saw a consultant his attitude was one of total dismissal. He told her to go away and come back when she was married and she felt that not only was she being ignored but also that he was dismissing her life. There were other, similar experiences in life and she remembers being told by a GP, a nurse, her family and others to 'wait until you get older – you don't know your own mind', attitudes which she described as astonishing. A friend with two children appeared to be cross after Anne D. attempted to discuss her ideas, and so she did not broach the subject with anyone else as she hated the feeling of having to justify and explain. Undeterred, she approached a Marie Stopes clinic in the north of England and, although she was quickly given a date for the operation, she was amazed at her complex reaction to this news. She felt that she 'had won' but describes her emotional reaction as one of loss and needing to acknowledge, mark and grieve for her 'soon-to-be-gone-fertility', despite definitely not wanting children in her life and feeling that she wanted to remain true to herself. The operation was arranged and carried out within three months of her application when she was 28. Anne D. now feels in control of this part of her life, and has no regrets at all.

Christine, from Dorset, aged 44: Christine is white, English and describes herself as a 'serial monogamist'. She finds living with people an intolerable strain and lives alone with her cat and dog. She is the eldest child with two brothers and is nominally Church of England but neither attends church nor practises any religion. She works full-time.

Christine's mind has always been made up about not having children, she has never felt any pressure and has always made her own decisions. She says that when she was younger she had no idea that getting pregnant was so easy, and her contraceptive practice before the age of 19 was 'either Durex or potluck!'. She tried using the cap, which 'didn't fit properly, then the coil which was agony'. After taking the Pill for some time she gave up because she felt permanently ill and it caused the unpleasant side effect of creating skin pigmentation patches which resulted in people telling her that she had 'dirty marks' on her face making her look as though she 'had a moustache!'. Christine has had four pregnancies, despite attempting to be careful in using contraceptives. She was first pregnant at the age of 19 and felt absolutely desperate but was helped then, and twice subsequently, by the British Pregnancy Advisory Service. On the third occasion Christine asked about sterilization but was told that it would not even be considered in one so young; she was then 32 and was advised that when she met the right man she would want a child. The sterilization was arranged by BPAS and carried out when she was 33 at the same time as her fourth abortion. Had she needed to discuss her plans with anyone she feels that she would have received support but did not seek any type of formal counselling as she was certain about the decision. Christine is aware that other women are puzzled by her childfree lifestyle and that they feel sorry for her, believing that she is naturally sterile. She is absolutely delighted at no longer needing to worry about getting pregnant and has never regretted either the decision or the operation.

Helen, from Kent, aged 38: Helen is white, Scottish and has had sexual relationships with both women and men, although she says that she 'dislikes the whole binary notion'. If pressed, she would say that she is heterosexual. Helen is divorced and through circumstance rather than choice has been celibate for over three years. She has an older brother and is spiritual rather than religious. Helen works for a health promotion unit as a sexual health specialist.

Helen has come to the understanding that a major reason for her not wanting children is her relationship with her mother who, she said, 'taught me to hate children'. She had been asking about sterilization since the age of 17 but was told by the family planning services that she was too young and would change her mind. She has not been pregnant nor had an abortion and her contraceptive history includes the Pill, coil and cap – none of which suited her – as well as having unprotected sex. Later, and after reading an article in a woman's magazine, she realized that she could again begin to seek sterilization and discussed her decision with husband and friends. The only counselling was a discussion of five minutes immediately before the operation, which she said 'was horrendous' as the initial anaesthetic did not work and she was given a general anaesthetic only when she screamed. The operation, which was paid for in instalments, was arranged through a Marie Stopes clinic. Helen was 23 when she was sterilized and says that if she had not seen the magazine article she would have continued with the Pill until she was in her thirties and then tried the NHS again. She feels angry that people felt that they had the right to hold strong opinions about her choice and that she was too young for sterilization, yet if a woman made a decision to have a child at 23 then that would be considered old enough. Helen thought about the operation every day for years and being sterilized is 'undoubtedly the greatest decision' in her life. Most people that she knows 'find it incomprehensible' that she opted for sterilization, but she was determined that she would not rely on less than one hundred per cent effective contraception throughout her fertile life. She says that she has no affinity with children at all and believes that she would have physically abused any child which she produced. Helen has never regretted being sterilized.

Ginny, from Devon, aged 35: Ginny is white, European and has several allergic conditions including asthma. When she was a young woman she had several lesbian relationships, is single and celibate now, but has been married. She is the eldest of four and was baptized into the Church of Jesus Christ of Latter Day Saints (Mormon Church). A volunteer worker with several women's groups, she is a secretary and not in paid employment at the time when she answered the advertisement.

Ginny was in her teens when she first knew that she did not want children. She did not want to be trapped, as she perceived her mother to be, by 'putting the children first'. Her Mormon Church upbringing told her that sex and pregnancy outside marriage is sinful, and abortion is murder. She used the Pill but reacted badly to it because of other medication that she was taking and says that she would have had an abortion if necessary because of an unwanted pregnancy. She believes that she has the right to make her own decisions in all matters and had her mother's support, although when the issue of her sterilization was discussed within her Church she 'felt total rejection' because of the belief that women's role is as wife and mother. Ginny's GP was very sympathetic to her enquiry about sterilization but she had a very negative experience with the NHS hospital to which she was referred. The operation was carried out when she was 32, one year after her initial request.

Ginny had feelings of total relief after the operation, no longer fears getting pregnant, nor any longer has any Pill-related problems with her medication.

Gillian, from Devon, aged 46: Gillian is white, British and has been married for twenty years. She is the elder of two children, with a younger brother who is married with three children, and although Church of England by faith was convent educated. Gillian is a trained nurse, has qualifications in yoga and counselling and works full-time with two part-time components to her work.

Gillian has never wanted children nor do babies appeal to her. She was definite from the age of 14 about remaining childfree and, when she married, she and her husband agreed that they neither wanted nor needed children. Apart from her extremely supportive GP, the decision was not discussed with anyone else. Her parents and friends were not happy when they found out and she says that there was some criticism. She could not take the Pill and, after failed contraception, she became pregnant during the waiting time for an NHS appointment. She consulted the BPAS and a termination and sterilization were carried out two weeks later: she was 26, three months after her marriage. Gillian wanted effective contraception and, apart from some post-operative problems, she has no regrets.

Gemma, from Glasgow, aged 34: Gemma is white, British, single and the youngest of two girls. Because of her premature birth she sustained cerebral palsy, with corrective surgery and therapy in infancy to minimize the effects. Her education was disrupted through the illness anorexia, and she has no formal qualifications. Gemma is committed to working with people and hopes to gain a regular position with a national advice agency.

Gemma says that she never had any maternal feelings. Post-anorectic problems and consequent difficulties with the Pill meant that she was uncertain about the pattern of her menstrual cycle and she even wondered whether she was infertile. She lived in fear of her body 'ambushing' her and it was this uncertainty which made her determined to apply for sterilization. She has identified that her rejection as a baby would make her a poor parent and has undergone therapy for her feelings of self-doubt and inadequacy. Gemma feels that she has begun to come to terms with the experiences of rape which resulted in pregnancy scares. Whilst waiting for her appointment for sterilization, she wanted to find out as much as possible about the procedure and read as much as she could find on the subject. Of the few people she told about her plans, some were sympathetic and supportive but others disapproved. The operation was straightforward, although Gemma was surprised and upset that she was given neither post-operative care nor advice which initially left her feeling vulnerable and anxious. She feels very positive about her decision to be sterilized and has no regrets.

Liz, from Hertfordshire, aged 43: Liz is white, British, heterosexual, and in a monogamous relationship. She was adopted, has an older brother who is the biological child of her adoptive parents, and describes herself as agnostic bordering on atheist. She is married for the second time, is a trained nurse and is manager of a Marie Stopes clinic.

Liz feels that she did not make a conscious decision to remain childfree but 'had always known' from her teenage years that she did not want children. Babies and small children leave her cold and she finds them intensely noisy and irritating. She questions 'whether selfish' is an appropriate word to use about being childfree and believes there are many selfish reasons for having children. She has observed that friends' needs 'are totally subjugated' by the needs of their families and she intends to live her own life rather than reliving and repeating parts which are in the past. When she was 17 and using no form of contraception she had an unplanned pregnancy. She reacted 'with extreme panic' and opted for termination which she has never regretted, knowing that it was the right decision for her. Liz used the Pill after that which she found suitable, but did not want to use it long-term, and her decision to be sterilized was made entirely independently of any relationship and to ensure that there could be no conflict about potential motherhood with any future partner. She had some discussion with friends who were, on the whole, supportive. She did not seek counselling as she was entirely comfortable with her decision. The waiting time after approaching the consultant was only a matter of weeks and was carried out in an NHS hospital when she was 30. Liz says emphatically that she has 'never ever had any regrets' about her decision.

Clare, from Cambridgeshire, aged 51: Clare is white, Anglo-Saxon, identifies as lesbian and is generally well. She is the elder of two with an adopted sister ten years younger, describing herself as agnostic, bordering on atheist. Clare was married for ten years and since her divorce has lived for fourteen years in a committed lesbian relationship. She is an NHS trained professional and works part-time in the NHS and part-time as a counsellor in private practice.

Clare recalls that, when she was 10 the adoption of her sister probably had an effect upon the way that she viewed babies and children. Until that age she was an only child, and has since realized that she made demands of her parents for a baby sister when what she really wanted was a playmate. The resulting reality of 'a squawking baby' restricted her activities. Clare feared unplanned pregnancy and her early sexual experiences resulted in failed contraception and a pregnancy scare. If necessary, she would have sought an abortion because, at that time, there was no morning-after pill. Remaining childfree was a condition of married life which she made clear when she accepted the proposal of marriage, despite being aware of the expectation of others, especially her mother-in-law, that she would have children. Clare participated in a medical trial on women's experiences of PMT conducted by a big training hospital and attributed feeling unwell to the Pill although, in retrospect, she feels that she 'didn't trust it'. She was unaware that counselling services existed at the time she was thinking about sterilization, which was also around the time when she was considering her sexuality. During the PMT trial she discussed the option of sterilization at the same hospital which then agreed to consider her application. She did not use her GP for referral but thinks it likely that the hospital informed him and the operation was carried out when she was 33. She recalls feeling that the ward medical staff regarded her as too young to undergo sterilization. Clare experienced some post-operative pain from adhesions, but has had no regrets about her decision, only feelings of relief.

Lesley, from Derbyshire, aged 42: Lesley is English, white, and describes herself as heterosexual. The younger of two, she has an older brother, and does not practise any religion. She has been divorced and her second husband has two children from his previous marriage. Lesley works on the factory floor of a large car manufacturing plant.

Lesley cannot recall any early pressures on her to become a mother although, as she grew older, she was aware that her mother wanted to be a grandmother. She and her first husband shared a great interest in sport and the issue of having children did not arise in that marriage, although she is sure that her Catholic mother-in-law would soon have begun to put pressure on her. Lesley relied on condoms as a teenager then, during the short period immediately before her second marriage, she had an unplanned pregnancy and sought an abortion. She recalls the discussion about sterilization with her GP as being quite factual and non-judgemental but, as she was only 27 and without children, he said she would not even be considered by the NHS and the application would be a complete waste of time. The Pill suited her reasonably well but the pregnancy scare was the deciding factor in knowing that she did not want children. She thinks that she gleaned information about sterilization by word-of-mouth from her all-female work environment. There was no counselling but she did have some discussions with her workmates, some of whom were supportive, although others were critical. At 28, in a private consultation, the gynaecologist 'asked very few personal questions' before moving quickly on to the method of payment. The operation was carried out within a month, she thinks by cauterization. Lesley has no regrets or doubts that her decision was right for her. She believes that if she had not had a scare and opted for sterilization when she was in her twenties, she would have reached the same decision in her late thirties to give her body a rest from the Pill.

Emma, from West Yorkshire, aged 24: Emma has known since the age of 16 that she does not want children and reflects that, in part, her certainty may stem from living in a series of children's homes with her parents who worked in them. From a loving and supportive background herself, she was exposed to the distress and emotional trauma of children whose parents did not want them or who abused and abandoned them. Because of this early awareness of the cruelty of some parents towards their own children, she is amazed and feels bitter that it is she who must account for her choice and decision to remain childfree. After contraceptive failure Emma underwent an abortion, which she found traumatic and distressing, later experiencing sadness, anger and guilt, feelings which she took to counselling.

Emma's early enquiries and requests for sterilization were dismissed and trivialized but as she grew older she was taken more seriously, although she found it difficult to sustain her determination in the face of negative and unhelpful responses. Initially she was unable to afford the fee for the Marie Stopes clinic, which includes counselling and consultation prior to the operation, and was astonished that her age was as much a factor for refusal by Marie Stopes as when she was exploring opportunities in the NHS. The comments and questions were identical, being that she might change her mind, or might meet someone, and that she had not had much life experience. Emma is a committed feminist and aware of the control held over her by those in the medical profession. She is angry that it is usually men, who can neither conceive nor understand women's lived experiences of their fertility, who hold the ultimate decision-making powers about women's choices. Emma resigned herself to having to wait, but one of her applications was successful, and she was sterilized at the age of 24 during the summer of 1997.

Jane, from East London, aged 59: Jane went almost to the end of her fertile years before considering seriously whether or not she wanted a child. She explored that question with a counsellor and was supported in finding the answer from within herself. She became a mother ten months later.

Jane realized that emotionally she had always wanted a child but that cognitively she always allowed her 'rational and sensible side to dom-inate'. At two previous points in her life she realized that she had allowed herself to be talked out of the idea of motherhood; in her thirties, she rationalized that she was the spouse in permanent work and again, in her early forties, was told and agreed that her age was against her. She reflects that it probably felt selfish as it was a decision which would be entirely for her. Her husband, previously married with children, realized that she needed to reach a resolve, so encouraged her to make a decision which he would fully support. She visited a counsellor feeling that she would experience 'a non-biased view'. Almost immediately, she realized that she already had the answer to her question, came off the Pill and was pregnant immediately. Jane feels that she was right to postpone her decision until she 'knew herself better' and now cannot imagine being without her son.

In the chapters ahead

This book explores the diverse reasons why an increasing number of women who are childfree by choice are going on to demonstrate their personal commitment to a childfree lifestyle by opting for sterilization. Through a consideration of the stories of 23 childfree sterilized women in Britain, and from a feminist research perspective, the study addresses the notion that there are continuous inexorable demands on all women to accept that motherhood is a blessed, assured and inevitable state. The study draws attention to the small number of women who resist the pressure to become mothers, confronting established medical opinion which refuses to accept that there are women who do not want children: women who, for their own reasons and in their own interests, use sterilization as their chosen method of ensuring that they remain child-free. Their stories illustrate aspects of the contemporary challenges to an assumption of biology as destiny or beliefs in an inherent, biological motherhood instinct.

Throughout the book I have attempted to represent the experiences and feelings of the women who shared their stories with me. Wherever possible I use their words to illustrate the more theoretical aspects of this study, particularly where it is clear that women's experiences offer a direct challenge to some (usually medical) 'received wisdom'. It is sobering to see how often this occurs, especially during their applications for sterilization, when they report that the reasons that they offer for making the decision to be sterilized are trivialized, dismissed or reinterpreted by doctors or consultants.

The previous section has presented the background to the book and personal rationale for the study and for using feminist research methods to facilitate hearing the voice of childfree sterilized women. The following section contained the 'profiles' which tell the women's stories. These were created from their diaries and interviews and introduced the women who participated in the study.

Chapter 1 addresses the complex issues surrounding womanhood and motherhood for women and, according to some research, the collapsing together of the two meanings. The diverse ways in which the contested area of gendering of the individual occurs are addressed and how women are subject to messages which point them in the direction of motherhood and their role as future carers, especially what has been described as the compulsory nature of heterosexuality. Biology as destiny and the influences of nurturing and socialization are considered and contrasted, as is the primary question of how it is some women say that they have no maternal feelings when the majority of other women anticipate and eagerly await the birth of children and the state of motherhood. Anthropological, cultural and psychological studies highlight the diversity of ways in which womanhood and motherhood are synonymous, and cultural beliefs of what it is to be a woman are considered. Also examined are the pressure and prejudice faced by women who are involuntarily childless, and the messages that are sent by this to any woman who contemplates remaining childfree. The unresolved issue of women's control of their own fertility draws this chapter to a close.

Chapter 2 opens with a brief historical account of contraception, birth control and family planning, including abortion and infanticide, and explores the influence of the eugenics movement in the UK and parallel birth control and family planning developments and movements in America. The development of barrier, IUD and chemical methods is examined from the 1930s, through the so-called 'sexual revolution' of the 1960s, and up to the present day: feminist critical comment on this era is part of this chapter. The control of women's reproduction through patriarchal systems (for example, the various religious and Church canon and diktats, through legislation and, with regard to this work, the medical profession) is also addressed with attention drawn to the effects of contemporary reproductive technologies. Comment and reports from two major world conferences which dealt with women's lives and freedoms are included and show the global nature of concerns and controversies about the place and role of women in society. There is a critical assessment of global debates on overpopulation and an examination of the assumptions made about the need for 'population control' programmes grounded in and working from a baseline of Western values and beliefs, utilizing a plethora of reproductive technologies, and imposing contraception and birth control measures in the majority world. Also suggested here is that sterilization is chosen by childfree women only when every month brings a dread of becoming pregnant and particularly after they have had a pregnancy scare; when they experience problems with contraception including failure; or when their doctors advise them to come off the Pill and use less reliable methods so as to give their bodies a rest. The assertion is made that doctors have ignored or failed to identify the two distinctly different groups of women who apply for sterilization: those who are mothers and who wish to cease using contraception so as to have no more children; and childfree women who say that they have 'always known' that they do not want children, who seek sterilization in order to give up obsolete 'monthly' contraception (in their terms), so as to have no children.

Chapters 1 and 2 focus on theoretical and literature contexts and the voice of the women, whilst present, supports and illustrates the themes rather than being predominant: subsequent chapters move the focus to the women themselves, their perceptions and experiences. Chapter 3 begins with an exploration of the stereotypes of women who remain childfree and, using the information gathered as part of the research from the women's own stories, addresses whether or not there are identifiable characteristics which set them apart from women who become mothers. It is identified that the only characteristic which appears to link them is that most assert that they had 'always known' that they did not want children. Their individual decisions and journey towards sterilization are charted and they emerge as women who had carefully and conscientiously attempted to avoid pregnancy by making use of the variety of contraceptive provision currently available. They describe their disappointment and dissatisfaction with the effectiveness or safety of monthly contraceptive measures and how they lived in fear of unplanned and unwanted pregnancies. The assertion is made that 'having' a child does not necessarily mean 'wanting' a child and there is a critical assessment of Adrienne Rich's notion of 'motherhood continuum'. The hostility directed towards them and a feeling of being considered to be not 'real' women is portrayed by the diarists, as are their own reasons for identifying elective sterilization as the most permanent way of ensuring that they would remain childfree for life and the details of the action that they took on the way to being sterilized.

Chapter 4 sets out and examines the major issues relating to the process of the women choosing to remain without children and making the decision to be sterilized. The women diarists give their personal accounts of these stages and reflect on how and when they knew they did not want children, recalling the period prior to making the decision including: which contraceptive methods had been used; whether any identified major events (such as a scare or a pregnancy, or medical advice to come off the Pill) acted as a catalyst to dissatisfaction with contraception; any important stages in the process of exploring the options and considering the implications of ceasing to use method contraceptives; then how they reached the decision to apply for sterilization. The individual stories of the women's personal determination to pursue elective sterilization is the major theme, focusing on the practical problems and barriers encountered by the women in opting for sterilization, including references to other interviews with medical specialists and pregnancy advisory practitioners. The women describe how they discovered the necessary advice and information to assist them in making their application. This part also examines how highly charged emotional issues are viewed and dealt with by the medical services, and how doctors and counsellors have diverse interpretations of the purpose and practice of counselling; and the women report on the prejudices and barriers they encountered from doctors and consultants, or other advisory services.

Chapter 5 examines the practical aspects of sterilization, the methods used and the aftermath of the operation. The women describe the formalities of the process leading up to the procedure and reflect on their perceptions and experiences of how they were treated in the hospitals or clinics. Sterilization as a positive choice is emphasized through the comments of the diarists and they also highlight the perceived need to prepare a 'plausible' story which would satisfy the consultant because of fear of further refusal. The experience of being sterilized is described and the period after sterilization examined for relief and regret. Also considered here is the medical view that many sterilized women regret having had the operation and request reversal, whilst the study establishes that 22 of the 23 childfree sterilized women had no regrets and would not consider having the procedure reversed. The study shows that the traditional view is based on the limited data available, which mainly relates to reversals on women who have already had children, thus presenting a strong challenge to the reasons given by doctors and consultants for refusing or postponing sterilization. It is suggested that the medical view of childfree women who apply for sterilization is often based on the unresearched, and therefore untested, belief or assumption that childfree women will change their minds and will inevitably apply for reversal.

The Conclusion draws together the main points of the book, emphasizing that many women do not easily conform to the ideology that every woman can be positioned as 'some-kind-of-mother', and proposes a set of five important preconditions which would enable women to be able to consider remaining childfree, to cease using contraception 'by the month' and to opt for sterilization. It is proposed that, even with maximum information and choice, the majority of women will continue to wish to have a child or children and that most will go on to do so. Even so, it is asserted that a minority of women act on their choice to remain without children, and elective sterilization may be the choice of an even smaller number of these childfree women. The suggestion is that there will be a future softening of current prejudices and disapproving social attitudes and that this in turn will influence and affect the medical world. Further developments and advances in contraceptive methods will provide the context for an increasing acknowledgement of the potential of elective sterilization for permanently preventing, rather than postponing, motherhood, although not all of the medical and social effects of reproductive technology will be welcomed. It is suggested that the decision not to have children will come to be seen as a valid choice and will be viewed less negatively in future as more women make clear their intention to remain childfree so that, stripped of the disapproval it currently attracts, elective sterilization may be an addition to the range of contraceptive provision currently available to British women.

Notes

1. When I eventually did have sight of my medical records I saw that the letter said;

> Thank you for asking me to see this 30 year old lady. As she is divorced I would not advise tubal ligation here. She was not at all pleased to hear this. She will be coming to see you quite shortly. I offered a gynaecological assessment but she did not wish this to be done. (26 January 1978)

2. With few exceptions, the women in this study do not describe themselves as feminists. Their diaries and the follow-up interviews show that most were not involved in nor more than vaguely aware of the struggle engaged in by second-wave feminists for women's domestic and reproductive rights. Instead, years of grappling with increasingly irrelevant contraceptive methods precipitated their active and vigorous pursuit of sterilization as their answer to remaining free from fear of unwanted pregnancy. Whereas feminists continue to assert as a feminist ideal that feminism does not seek to free women from motherhood but is concerned to free them from the oppressive conditions which accompany motherhood (Richardson, 1993), the women in this study did not contemplate any lifestyle which included the state of motherhood, regardless of the conditions attached to it.

3. Patriarchy is a term contested within feminist theories (and refused by some writers: Sheila Rowbotham (1981), for example) with diverse critiques from Marxist and radical feminists' perspectives and from Black feminist writers. I felt that the term would be useful within the study but wanted to avoid suggesting that patriarchy as a system provides the only reason that women and men occupy different positions in society. Within the context of this study a difference of power emerged in the reported relationships between the women and the doctors and specialists (both female and male) whom they encountered, and this occurred and was located in the UK medical system. There were a number of references to patriarchy within the medical sociology texts that I was using which highlighted aspects of the power imbalance which had been identified in the diaries and during the interviews with the women (for example: Turner, 1987, Ch. 5, 'Women's complaints: patriarchy and illness'; Brown (ed.), 1996, various authors, but especially Susan Bell, 'Political gynecology'; Maureen Porter, Ch. 8, 'Professional-client relationships and women's reproductive health care', in Cunningham-Burley and McKeganey, 1990; Mary James, Ch. 6 'Hysteria', in Seale and Pattison, 1994 (2nd edn.) and Nicky Hart, 1985, writes about 'patriarchal capitalism'). Rosalind Pollack Petchesky, in her

report on the Cairo Conference (International Conference on Population and Development, 1994) wrote 'Contrary to the insistence of the Vatican and other fundamentalists on a single, universally normative family structure (the patriarchal, conjugal, heterosexual kind) . . . ' (Petchesky, 1995).

Seeking definitions of the term was useful: Maggie Humm (1989) writes; 'Patriarchy has power from men's greater access to and mediation of the resources and rewards of authority structures inside and outside the home'; and Sylvia Walby (1990) opens her chapter on 'Culture' thus: 'Ideas about masculinity and femininity are to be found in all areas of social relations; they are part of the actions which go to make up the patriarchal structures'. Women in this study encountered resistance to their requests for sterilization as a consequence of engaging in 'social relations' within these 'authority structures'. My references to patriarchal systems, patriarchal structures, patriarchal attitudes or other phrases which qualify the word patriarchy, use the word in the spirit of its use by other writers as well as consciously directing a narrow focus onto the medical world.

Womanhood and Motherhood

I am very interested in what are the social and psychological factors that cause some of us to be so sure about the choice to be childfree when all the pressure is to have children. (Jill)

At every level of social and cultural interaction girls and women are exposed to assumptions and expectations that all women will become mothers. Although this is traditionally presented as normal and natural, media and research reports in the mid-1990s highlighted and uncovered an emerging trend. There are indications that, despite society's emphasis on all things maternal some women no longer accept the inevitability of motherhood and have moved beyond thinking about when to have a baby and onto considering whether they want to become mothers at all.

Motherhood has a social and compulsory aspect ensuring that women's choices are highly circumscribed (Hanmer, 1993). Even when parents have high ambitions for their children's education and eventual successful careers, there is likely to be an underlying expectation – especially for girls – that marriage or a happy partnership and parenthood will form some part of the future for their children, and grandparenthood for themselves. Traditionally, girls are presented with an idealized image of themselves as future mothers with the result that, for many girls, 'motherhood remains one of the most positive aspects of the feminine role' (Sharpe, 1976). From the earliest days of infancy, throughout childhood and into their maturity, females are prepared not only for womanhood but also for motherhood, and in most cultures girls are perceived as and considered to be potential mothers even though, in general, young women remain unaware of the oppressive conditions attached to the role of wife and mother. As 'mother' is a socially constructed role it cannot be seen as 'natural' (Nicolson, in Richardson and Robinson, 1993), yet unlike many other cultural roles, titles or status (wife, teacher, working-class) which may change, be discarded or cease to exist, women's experience of giving birth is irreversible. It seems that when a baby is born, also a mother is created.

The first name that every baby is given at birth is the one relating to biology; girl or boy, female or male. There are only two sexes at this early, crucial birth period: no other categories are available or possible. Until very recently, if there was immediate difficulty in identifying the sex of a baby born with what are considered to be genital abnormalities, some one of the birth attendants – usually a doctor – would pronounce which of the two sexes was most likely to describe the child. Important work carried out in the USA[1] appeared to show that, in such instances, even where a female child was incorrectly ascribed at birth, corrective gender-socialization by parents and within the culture tended to reverse or at least balance out early tendencies towards 'male' behaviour. If the mistake was recognized and corrected the child could adapt to the new sex and begin to act in appropriate gender-behaviour ways without overtly serious consequences. However, it was essential that this happened before the age of 2 and preferably by the age of eighteen months, otherwise it would prove extremely difficult to re-educate the child (in Davenport, 1988). Gender identity – the perception of the self as being male or female – depends on whether a child has been reared as a girl or as a boy 'even when this is in contrast to its biological sex' (Brierley, 1987). The opportunity to utilize contemporary genetic testing in order to establish sex via the chromosome make-up may prevent future wrong-sexing at birth, but changing the official sex must happen very quickly in a child's life if it is to be effective.

There is continuing and intense debate and disagreement about the dominant influences of the nature or nurture aspects of child development, with social learning theories proposing that children learn their gender roles through a combination of being taught and directed by parents towards what it is to be a girl or a boy and also by observing significant models around them. A number of anthropological studies have highlighted that there is such a variation between cultures, between peoples and even between individuals of the same sex, that gender behaviour is unlikely to have a biological basis and is much more likely to be as a result of parental and cultural expectations of appropriate female or male behaviour (Mead, 1935 and 1949; Lewis and Rosenblum, 1979; Taylor, 1996). The biological theories of gender are based on arguments which attempt to show that there are significant differences in the attitudes and behaviour of females and males and that these differences are instincts which are genetically transmitted (Freud, 1905; Bowlby, 1965), although there has been some shifting in ground, away from the polarization of either nature or nurture. A common view is now that, even though females and males do have obvious biological differences and a differential hormonal balance – which may even be linked to certain identifiably different kinds of behaviour between the sexes – this does not mean that aspects of the socialization process cannot override what in the past have been considered to be immutable biological urges (Davenport, 1988). One of these urges was believed to be a woman's impetus towards motherhood. This study and others like it present strong challenges to such an assumption.

The process of gender internalization (Golombok and Fivush, 1994) begins in infancy and continues through childhood and adolescence. Feminist research and childhood studies show that babies are treated in significantly different ways depending on their sex, and observations of the physical handling of babies and adults' choices of what are considered to be appropriate gifts and toys show that gender is perceived to be a major feature of the developing child (Lewis and Rosenblum, 1979). Various studies in the field of social learning theory and developmental psychology show that most children begin to identify what sex they are from at approximately eighteen months of age (Bem, 1974; Bandura, 1977; Bleir, 1984; Brierley, 1987; Golombok and Fivush, 1994), although this appears to remain a rather loose and flexible area of their knowledge for several years more. Most female young children know, for example, that they are 'a girl' and show an ability to identify other girls or boys as such quite often from the clues of hair and clothes, but in early childhood they believe that when they grow up they could become the opposite sex if they changed their appearance. Girls maintain this flexibility about the possibilities of changing gender for longer than boys and will imitate male role models to a greater extent than boys will imitate female role models and, although girls know more about gender than do boys, boys are more sex-typed than are girls.

It is simply more acceptable for girls to engage in cross-sex-typed behaviors, such as playing with cars and trucks, than for boys to engage in cross-sex-typed behaviors, such as playing with baby dolls and dressing up. There is no simple explanation for this. But certainly males and, by extension, stereotypically male behaviors [sic] are seen more positively in our culture. And males hold more power than females. Therefore, it is more advantageous for females to know about males than it is for males to know about females. (Golombok and Fivush, 1994, 228)

There are clearly different gender expectations for even the very youngest children and parents tend to encourage and reinforce the gendered behaviour of daughters and sons. In their belief that sex-role behaviours are linked to sexuality, most parents in traditional families fear that their children will become homosexual if they do not act in sex-role appropriate ways (Richardson, 1988), although adults' efforts aimed at ensuring that children will develop as heterosexual have no guarantee of success (Butler, 1990; Brooks, 1997). Whilst the effects of socialization and gendering are not identical for every individual, feminists have advanced the case that gender identity is fixed through the internalization of a culturally shaped set of attributes and behaviours which are presented as normal and appropriate for women and men and which are the opposite of each other (de Beauvoir, 1953; Firestone, 1970; Millett, 1970; Chodorow, 1978; O'Brien, 1983; Golombok and Fivush, 1994).[2] Unless challenged and contested by the individual (Bailey, 1993, in Brooks, 1997), this continuous process makes gender a major part of early consciousness. Once fully in place, usually by the age of 5, it is thought to be almost impossible to unlearn.

With the 'nature or nurture' debate continuing to rage, it has been fuelled by strong representations from researchers with a leaning towards sociobiology. The recurring descriptive term 'biology as destiny', and references to an essential 'mothering instinct', seems to indicate an often unconscious and generally unchallenged belief that all women want and need children and have an inherent impulse towards conception and, ultimately, motherhood. Modern variants of such notions pop up under a sociobiology heading which presents so-called evidence not only that certain behaviours differ according to sex as a result of being genetically programmed but also that the system of patriarchy is an inevitable result of male dominance (Goldberg, 1979). More recent arguments purport to provide scientific evidence to support the inevitability of women's subordination and male dominance: that is, that brain differences between female and male is to be found in their respective 'wiring'.[3] These sorts of arguments have tremendous currency as they mesh with the dominant ideas of Western societies and a branch of scientific inquiry which seeks proof (currently through genetic research) that gender characterizations and divisions are natural.

Recent research suggests that much of the 'nervous wiring' of the human brain takes place as a result of the learning process during early life (Edelman, 1990, in Taylor, 1996), and a variety of theories have been advanced in attempts to justify inequalities between the sexes. For example, it is suggested that women have a smaller brain (there were media reports during 1997 of an amazing pregnancy-induced 'shrinking brain'); the Victorians believed that women should avoid intellectual work because of the taxing effect on their brains which would result in their succumbing to 'the vapours', or they would become hysterical and overwrought. Such arguments echo, in part, a plethora of 'logical reasons' used in the nineteenth century to attempt to justify the exclusion of women from higher education and the professions (Sayers, 1982; Acker, 1994), and, if no other reason was found to be plausible, the capacity for childbearing and nurturing itself was seen as sufficient cause for women's inferiority (Charles, 1993).[4]

There are, however, robust challenges and resistance to such essentialist proposals. Describing as 'nonsense' the Western habit of discounting the impact of culture during early life, archaeologist Timothy Taylor argues that babies are treated as male or female from birth and are, therefore, far from the completely natural beings 'from whose behaviour general principle of sexual difference can be inferred' (Taylor, 1996). Babies and young children in any society are reared by adults who overtly and unconsciously expose the developing individual to close contact with all of the dominant philosophies and principles held to be real, true, normal and deemed vital to the health, well-being and successful smooth running of the culture. Crucial structures such as the family, law and the educational process may present serious conflicts for those who do not comply with cultural beliefs, morals and standards, and in most societies and cultures it is considered normal and natural for individuals to be heterosexual, to marry and for women to achieve motherhood.

Margaret Mead (1949) pointed out that, as social conditions change, each culture perceives mothering and motherhood in different ways, attributing and expecting different behaviours, attitudes and feelings from women who are mothers (in Humm, 1989) with the distinct tendency for the meaning and understanding of 'woman' and 'mother' to collapse together (Petchesky, 1980; Morell, 1994). Regardless of the reproductive potential or otherwise of her male partner, in some cultures a woman has a designated low status if she is perceived as barren or if she is 'only' able to bear female babies. Although in global terms children are seen as a valuable resource and their absence from the lives of married adults is viewed as a personal and social tragedy, for the majority of women in the world there is no opting-out of motherhood. Nor is there is much realizable choice about whether or not to have a child. The appropriate time for socially approved sexual activity for women and consequent motherhood is usually also carefully monitored and often will be supported by expectations of chastity and virginity and the careful supervision and chaperoning of unmarried girls until they are married.

The role of women as carers, and the social and cultural range of choices available to women when they consider becoming mothers (or when facing the unplanned prospect of motherhood), has been a major area of research and writing for feminists of all theoretical perspectives. A major strand of feminist theory[5] considered the patriarchal and political dimension of motherhood to be primary, with a historical dependency on men, especially during pregnancy and child-rearing, which has contributed to women's oppression. Women's reproductive role, therefore, became identified within many feminist theories as the primary cause of male domination serving to maintain women's subservience to men. Shulamith Firestone (1970) asserted that women are handicapped by their role as reproducers and claimed that childbearing and women's central role in child-rearing are at the heart of the most fundamental divide in society: the gendered division between women and men. She posited that motherhood is indicative of women's unique and special value but is utilized as a form of oppression by powerful patriarchal systems and concluded that concepts of 'motherhood' and 'freedom' are diametrically opposed. Firestone presented what she understood to be fundamental, if not immutable, facts, the first of which stemmed from her commitment to biological essentialism and her belief that reproductive biology was the origin of a continuing oppression of women rather than any sudden patriarchal revolution. Thus, prior to contemporary methods of birth control, women's biology (pregnancies, childbirth and the care of infants) created women's dependency on males for physical survival.

This argument has been taken up and challenged by many feminists and has been rejected by most (Jackson *et al.*, 1993), although it is difficult not to admire the passion which is at the heart of Firestone's 'bold and revolutionary text' (Stacey, in Richardson and Robinson, 1993). A useful analysis of Firestone's argument that biology is at the heart of the sexual division of labour asserts that women's subordination to men and the 'tyranny of their reproductive biology' (Shilling, 1993) can be broken only through new reproductive technologies. Other feminists focus on the mothering ideology present within all societies which may be in the form of maternal thinking (Ruddick, 1982) or as a 'feminist discourse which is embedded with maternal values and ways of seeing' (Humm, 1989). The mythological, mysterious and powerful distinction accorded to all women in systems informed by patriarchal notions becomes a complex and contradictory discourse of womanhood/ motherhood, with women's choices constrained by expectations that they will aspire to mother, whether or not they go on to do so (Nicolson, in Richardson and Robinson, 1993).[6] This view represents the particular struggle for women who encounter a '"shifting terrain" on their way to claiming a personhood' (Hanmer, in Richardson and Robinson, 1993) and is indicative of the problems encountered in challenging definitions of correct or appropriate behaviour for women, and assumptions and beliefs about what constitutes a real or truly feminine woman.[7]

The ideas and beliefs which any society holds in its definition and social meaning of motherhood direct attention towards the place and role of women: that is, who, what and how they are. As the words woman and mother become synonymous, womanhood collapses into motherhood with the potential problems of 'turning all women into some-kind-of-mother' (Morell, 1994) and placing all women at some point along a 'motherhood continuum' (Rich, 1976). If woman and mother are perceived as meaning the same thing, then those women who reject motherhood and do not have children may become the target of disapproval and censure, experiencing problems about their place in society. When it is normal for all women to be mothers then women who decide not to have children stand out as oddities. Women with children and childfree women then occupy different places within society and, if not directly in opposition to each other, are at least uneasily aware of the gulf which separates them.

Motherhood boundaries

> To choose to have a child as a single woman or a lesbian is still to invite all the Furies that society can loose upon us. (Dowrick and Grundberg, 1980, 9)

The wealth of literature on mothering and motherhood highlights that women who want and have children are seen as normal. Childfree women's association with womanhood is questioned, social and cultural norms are threatened and this 'creates hierarchies among women based on reproductive difference', with motherhood and motherliness not just social roles and relationships but a state of being (Morell, 1994). In many cultures this idea is seen to be the primary purpose of a woman's life so that the meanings of woman and mother collapse together into 'maternalism' (Petchesky, 1980). Women are expected to experience motherhood unambivalently and are seen primarily as mothers; 'in accordance with patriarchal values, [a] "non-mothering" woman is seen as deviant' (Rich, 1976).

Compulsory heterosexuality (Rich, 1980) and the regulation of women's sexual behaviour and fertility are positioned within marriage and the family and promoted 'as the model for other social institutions of a sexual norm' (Humm, 1989), with the norm for sexual activity taken to be heterosexual (Wilkinson and Kitzinger, 1993). Disapproval of homosexual and lesbian partnerships is deeply embedded in notions of what is natural, and lesbian writers argued in the 1970s that heterosexuality is a social institution which underpins women's oppression (Humm, 1989). To be married, or in a sexual relationship, draws attention to the expected procreative capacity of the couple. Biblical references are invoked even more fiercely than for heterosexual behaviour and are often presented through a creationist belief that 'God created man and woman' with further emphasis by religious ministers and leaders that 'He' also created marriage for the direct purpose of producing children. That same-sex couples are vilified if they make known their intent to produce and raise a family is further testament to the essentialist nature of heterosexual coupledom.

Powerful beliefs and taboos surround the creation of life, and the control of an individual's sexual behaviour and reproduction features in many cultures. Notions of virginity and purity, chastity and virtue are closely aligned with the moral standards of cultures and societies by defining and monitoring sexual activity for all members, especially women. The sexual double standard is not a recent notion, nor is it culturally specific, and women who defy the taboos are castigated and often attract descriptive – usually pejorative – titles. Men who openly proclaim their level of heterosexual activity are considered to be behaving normally: similar behaviour in a woman is viewed as deviant, abnormal and even dangerous, for themselves, for their male partners and for society in general (de Beauvoir, 1953; Greer, 1970; Bryson, 1992). Women's sexual behaviour has until very recently been perceived and defined as mainly reproductive rather than recreative, so that women who remain unmarried, or who engage in and appear to enjoy sex outside a socially recognized and approved relationship, are very quickly made aware of society's disapproval.

In many cultures, especially Judaeo-Christian based, women tend to be viewed and positioned as either Madonna or Whore and there is a wealth of descriptive words for women (but seldom for men) who are seen to stray even slightly outside these narrow boundaries. A further dimension of such restrictive regulation is the 'gatekeeper' role, whereby women are expected to control and take responsibility for their own as well as men's sexual behaviour, in addition to birth control measures traditionally assumed to be the woman's responsibility (Richardson, in Richardson and Robinson 1993).

In the West, with only relatively recent awareness, knowledge and use of contraceptive methods, women who engage in heterosexual sex and who wish to avoid unwanted pregnancies are confronted with several possibilities: not taking contraceptive precautions at all, thus risking pregnancy; using contraception for family planning then ceasing when attempting to conceive; or taking all appropriate measures to remain without children. It is this ongoing necessity for all women to monitor their bodies, and be constantly vigilant in order either to become pregnant or to prevent conception, that Adrienne Rich (1976) refers to in her notion of a motherhood continuum. Once a woman has been sterilized, however, it would seem that she has no place on this continuum. Even if she continues in any other role as carer her potential for motherhood, either real or symbolic, has ceased.

Despite the dismissive slight, that women who opt for sterilization hail from 'the wilder shores of the feminist movement' (Allen, 1985), the issue of reproductive rights is a central and hotly debated feminist consideration, with women's control of their own reproduction an agreed feminist goal. Elective sterilization is not new, although it is still very rare for women who have no children to make such a choice, so that, whilst some feminists view motherhood as a 'barbaric relic of a lower state of human development from which women can now be liberated' (Bryson, 1992), others believe that it exemplifies women's superior creativity and virtue. Stripped of negative meaning as a patriarchal institution, motherhood would be a joyful and transforming experience for women (Rich, 1976, in Humm, 1994) and society would benefit through the power of maternal energy (Gilman, 1911).

Regardless of any other divisions which exist between the various feminist perspectives, there is general agreement amongst feminists that control of their own reproduction is an essential feature of women's self-determination and 'the right to reproductive freedom must be a cornerstone of women's liberation' (Humm, 1989). Yet it remains the case, at the end of the second millennium, that there is nowhere in the world where women have gained anything approaching control over their own bodies nor have full reproductive rights been achieved.[8]

Notes

1. The main area of research on the effects of hormones on human gender roles was on women who had been prescribed a miscarriage-preventative drug containing androgens during pregnancy and had given birth to female children who looked as though they had male sex organs. The name and diagnosis given was that they were suffering from Androgenital Syndrome requiring genital-corrective surgery (in Davenport, 1988).
2. Postfeminist critiques contend that the notion of gender is itself socially constructed and insist that there must be a reconsideration of many areas of debate established during second-wave feminism particularly '[gender which] drew a distinction

between "sex" which was taken to be universal and biological, and "gender" which was understood as culturally variable' (Brooks, 1997). At this fundamental level 'gender differences between male and female roles are then seen as social rather than biological [and] are changeable by human agency'; the sociocultural and historical characteristics of both sex as a biological category as well as gender became a central issue in the debate (Bailey, 1993, in Brooks, 1997).

3. Popularized in, for example, *BrainSex* (Moir and Jessell, 1989) a book written by a geneticist and a journalist, and *The Sexual Brain* (LeVay, 1993).

4. Nickie Charles gives a particularly good account of the feminist challenge to sociobiology in Chapter 1, 'Theorising origins: biology versus culture', of her book *Gender Divisions and Social Change* (1993).

5. For example: Wollstonecraft, 1992 (1792); de Beauvoir, 1953 (1949); Firestone, 1970; Brownmiller, 1975; Gordon, 1976; Rich, 1976; Petchesky, 1980; Dally, 1982.

6. From the 1960s, the struggle for women's 'rights' including reproductive rights was a major focus for feminist writers who were developing and establishing many of the theories from which contemporary feminisms spring. In her study of the 'backlash' against feminism (1991), Susan Faludi includes a short section on the more recent work of those early, most influential, feminist thinkers and writers. Betty Friedan's 1981 book *The Second Stage* is described as being revisionist in its attack upon the modern feminist movement; Faludi says that Friedan was 'yanking out the stitches in her own handiwork'. Germaine Greer's 1984 *Sex and Destiny* is 'dour and deterministic', with the future outlook for sex being one where abstinence is the best form of birth control. Susan Brownmiller, who produced *Against Our Will: Men, Women, and Rape* (1975), praised as 'a meticulously documented historical analysis of sexual violence', re-emerged to write *Femininity*, which Faludi calls 'a fuzzy look at feminine behaviour through the ages'. Her critique compares the language of the 'New Right' – a 'pro-family' semantics trap – to the seeming back-pedalling of 'old-line feminists'. She contrasts this approach with that of Camille Paglia, hailed with glee and feted by the media as a 'new-style' feminist. Faludi, however, describes Paglia as 'an embittered anti-feminist academic' who, because of 'snubs' from female scholars, reacted by wreaking a revenge motivated by 'spite'.

7. Femininity was presented by Freud as the normal state of womankind and the challenges to this are many and varied; indeed 'all the evidence goes to show that the "normal" woman is a somewhat rare phenomenon, and when we do come across her, it would seem that she does not stand out as a model of normality' (Lacan, 1975, in Mitchell and Rose, 1982). A contemporary definition of femininity may result in descriptions of an elegant woman or a nubile girl, scented, carefully made-up, dressed in a fashionable but not provocative way, demure but expectant of her future role as wife and (her highest ambition) mother. Some women may be mortified if they were to be accused of being unfeminine, but for others it may be a way to reclaim the self. I have always enjoyed Germaine Greer's attack on the falseness of femininity (from *The Female Eunuch*):

> So what's the beef? Maybe I couldn't make it. Maybe I don't have a pretty smile, good teeth, nice tits, long legs, a cheeky arse, a sexy voice . . . maybe I don't know how to handle men. Then again, maybe I'm sick of the masquerade. I'm sick of pretending eternal youth. I'm sick of belying my own intelligence, my own will, my own sex . . . I'm sick of being a transvestite. I refuse to be a female impersonator. I am a woman, not a castrate. (Greer, 1970, 61–2)

8. Globally, contraceptive commodities and services are controlled, held – and may also be withheld – within cultural systems which have beliefs and opinions about the status and place of women and the role of mother. At the end of the twentieth century, and after more than three decades of supposed sexual liberation, the struggle that women face in demanding reproductive rights continues to make news headlines. Abortion clinics in Britain are picketed and, in America, are bombed and attacked, sometimes resulting in the deaths of medical staff. Legislation is often used to support the witholding of information and services: putative fathers delay or attempt to prevent abortions, young Irish women are prevented from leaving their country to travel to mainland Britain for abortion and, as in the victory briefly won by Victoria Gillick in the 1980s, there are challenges to privacy when contraceptive information is sought by girls of under 16.

2

Population and Contraception, Past and Present

I don't have a child for my own selfish reasons. I haven't got the time, I haven't got the patience, and I don't want to waste my money on a child. On a larger scale I think that it would be the best thing for the planet if the human race died out because it is only us that trash it . . . so, I have a plethora of reasons why I don't want children but generally I don't think that as a species we should continue to procreate . . . (Linda L.)

We are now in the sixth mass extinction over the past 500 million years. Not because of meteorites, nor is it due to the Ice Ages, or the various other things which have been proposed as mechanisms for mass extinction. This mass extinction is due to us – you, and me. The World's population is increasing at an incredible rate: the degradation of our environment and the pollution are leading to inevitable species loss. (Professor Simon Conway Morris, 1996)

Reports from a variety of sources in the mid-1990s show that the population of the world grows annually by over 88 million. Population predictors show that a figure of over six billion is expected before the end of the twentieth century, an increase of 58 per cent since 1950.[1] The

United States population alone currently stands at 263 million and is added to by something like 2.5 million each year, making the US one of the world's fastest-growing industrialized nations. Conversely, in Britain over the last century the proportion of children in the population has declined, falling from a third to a fifth and, during the 1990s, the reported birth rate dropped below what has been considered as a 'replacement level' of 2.4, to 1.9 children in the 'average' family (World Health Organisation, 1995 figures). Given the many global concerns about overpopulation, fewer people being born would appear to be a reason for celebration rather than a cause for anxiety and yet this reported drop in the UK birth rate resulted in a flurry of concern that Britain is heading for a problem of underpopulation.

In the mid-nineteenth century the world population stood at one billion, doubled within a century, and the third billion was reached by 1950 with an average life expectancy of 35 years (Johnson, 1994). At the beginning of the 1990s the figure was nearing 5.3 billion: that is, five times as large as in 1798 when Thomas Malthus first wrote his essays in which he linked the rapid growth in population with poverty and starvation. In the developed world men live on average 72 years and women 78 but the global average life expectancy is far lower at just 55 years (Graham-Smith, 1994).

It is not easy to see an immediate connection between the fears expressed about underpopulation as an inevitable result of the Second World War, and reports of Britain's falling birth rate 50 years later. Post-war newspaper headlines reported on 'Empty Quivers',[2] and reporters carried out investigations into 'Homes without babies' (*Sunday Pictorial*, 1949). At the end of the twentieth century a proliferation of 'world-watch' organizations, environmental agencies, demographers and observers and commentators on global issues are emphasizing the pressures put on world resources by overpopulation[3] followed quickly by media articles with titles such as 'No kids on the block' (*Guardian*, 11 April 1995), 'Mum's not the word' (*Sunday Times*, 16 April 1995) and the more basic leader 'New breed of non-parents turns back on family way' (*Observer*, 16 April 1995). Media-focused scares such as this are not new, but they appear to be indicators of the strong feelings which are aroused when attention is drawn to childfree choices and lifestyles. A falling birth rate in the UK, a country which in common with other developed countries is a heavy consumer of global resources, would seem to be a trend to be welcomed and yet, as seen by the concern shown in the media, any change at any time is worthy of remark and investigation.

The announced drop in the British birth rate coincided with a report, quickly picked up by newspapers and other media, that the Family Policy Studies Centre was conducting a research project focusing on women's decision-making on motherhood (Condy, 1995). A radio programme debated the question, 'Do women have a moral duty to be mothers?' (*The Moral Maze*, Radio 4, June 1995), and lead articles appeared identifying that a few women had begun to assert their decision not to have children. Under the banner headline 'No Kids Please – We're Trendy' a popular daily newspaper announced that, after the Yuppies and the Dinkies 'now meet the PFA's: Pre-Family Adults' (*Daily Mirror* News Special, 7 June 1996), which highlighted what they reported to be a growing trend for a certain type of both men and women who seem reluctant to give up 'their self-indulgent life-styles'. Not everyone shared this concern. Under the headline, 'Give kids a wide birth' [*sic*], Fiona Webster offered her full support to the childfree 20- to 34-year-olds; 'Twenty per cent don't want children at all. Good for them. We should applaud their bravery, not condemn their selfishness. Having kids is still considered the norm' (*Daily Telegraph*, 14 June 1995)

The notion of choice in parenting is relatively new. Indeed, until the condom was refined during the 1930s and barrier methods were improved, the prevention of pregnancy was hazardous and chancy, despite zealous intervention and determination, and owed more to myth and so-called 'old wives' tales' than to knowledge and planning. Contraception has a recorded history in early Egypt, and in Roman times a number of methods were employed, including vinegar soaked sponges which were inserted into the vagina, indicating some awareness (although not necessarily by the user), or passed-on information, that an acid environment is hostile to sperm (Ariès, in de Beauvoir, 1953; Taylor, 1996). Other methods such as douching were also employed, often with the unfortunate effect of driving sperm even deeper, but the final solution was often a desperate attempt at abortion, resulting in haemorrhage, septicaemia and the deaths of both woman and unwanted foetus.

There is no record of contraceptive use in Europe up to the eighteenth century, although it is generally believed to have been practised (de Beauvoir, 1953) and there is nothing to show that notions of population control relating to overpopulation were prevalent prior to this, although there are well-documented attempts at genocide for political and racial or cultural reasons (Ariès, in de Beauvoir, 1953). The birth rate was not a matter publicly discussed or debated, nor is there evidence of pronouncements on what was considered to be an appropriate number of children for a woman to have. Historically, as in contemporary societies, it was only in the aftermath of invasions and wars that demands for higher birth rates were made, and replacement births, particularly of males for fighting, became urgent (Graham-Smith, 1994).

The term birth control is often used as though it were recently coined yet its practice was not fabricated by scientists or doctors but was invented by ordinary women as part of the folk culture of many early societies. If the community was nomadic, strategies would have included abstention, abortion and infanticide and none of these was considered to be either illegal or immoral (Seal, 1990), although there is a historic view of contraceptive use being suspected as a practice employed by prostitutes, or at least women of loose morals (de Beauvoir, 1953). A wide range of early contraceptive strategies was employed to ensure that birth rates did not threaten or overwhelm community resources, even one which demanded the use of honey mixed with crocodile dung from the banks of the Nile, a ubiquitous example appearing in a number of historical accounts (Wood and Suitters, 1970; Greer, 1984; Taylor, 1996, *inter alia*). Ever since they made the connection between intercourse and pregnancy, women have been trying to prevent unwelcome pregnancies and 'physicians have been prescribing potions, contraptions, herbs, and even incantations to help women achieve their goal (Fromer, 1983).

By the middle of the eighteenth century the world population was 771 million and increasing, although an individual's life expectancy of 22 years in AD 0 had risen only to 27 years by 1750 (Graham-Smith, 1994). Following the late seventeenth-century appearance of the 'science of demography' came the development of 'political arithmetic'. Birth and death rates were calculated and compared, and concerns began to be expressed about the means of subsistence and world potential for providing sufficient food and support to deal with increased populations (Livi-Bacci, 1992, in Graham-Smith, 1994). Thomas Malthus's constant theme was that populations will always outgrow the means of subsistence, yet despite this, and as a cleric, he did not approve of contraception, calling instead for sexual abstinence.[4] His later essays developed this theme and he advocated the 'preventive check' on population which, he believed, would be a consequence of people's self-restraint as they became better educated and more wealthy (Graham-Smith, 1994).

The social reformer and Chartist writer Francis Place understood that calls for such moral restraint were neither useful nor practical and, in the early nineteenth century, advocated instead the 'precautionary means' of withdrawal and sponges. In the wake of such publicity, many advocates, proponents and activists arose as champions of birth control. However, the moral climate was such that *Fruits of Philosophy*, a tract written by Charles Knowlton in 1841 and republished by Charles Bradlaugh and Annie Besant in 1877, was considered obscene and likely to deprave the morals of the general public, a pronouncement which resulted in their celebrated court appearances (Wood and Suitters, 1970). So as to further emphasize the outrage felt by the society at the time, a Dr Arthur Albutt was struck off the Medical Register in 1886 after publishing *The Wife's Handbook*, by any contemporary reasonable standards a sober and informative book intended to be helpful to women in labour and with advice on the aftercare of the baby.[5]

Women themselves have always taken steps to implement personal decisions about regulating their own bodies. In the past – as in many contemporary contexts – they would attempt to use often crude contraceptive methods in the first instance, abortion if pregnancy occurred and infanticide if other methods had failed or been prevented: by such means women were capable of limiting family size whether or not their actions were judged to be either moral or legal. The latter half of the nineteenth century was a period when issues relating to sexuality, reproduction and mothering were subjected to 'an intense legal gaze' (Smart, 1992) and a time when existing stringent sanctions on abortion were strengthened, with many further legislative attempts to curb the increased incidence of infanticide (Hoffer and Hull, 1981). This period was significant and marked 'a specific moment of struggle over the use of law to regulate the feminine body' (Smart, 1992).

That period of late nineteenth and early twentieth century also marked the struggle of the birth control pioneers against an ignorance which led to family poverty, misery and ill-health.[6] They fought against arguments designed to resist change and faced accusations ranging from encouraging promiscuity, distributing pornography and encouraging premarital sex, to being unpatriotic and flying in the face of God's will. Motherhood was lauded as the supreme role for women and, because children were gifts from God, it was promoted that contraceptives would be harmful to women's health (Suitters, 1973, in Huston, 1992). Fears voiced at that time and echoed today (Mass-Observation, 1942; Vatican encyclicals, *passim*; Smart, 1992) tie into beliefs that, because having children is what women do, contraceptive use would threaten not only marriage but also its main purpose – biological reproduction.

The rapid drop in family size is a feature of post-war Britain. Exhausted women, worn out at 40 by annual childbearing and written about with such passion, had inspired the work of early birth control pioneers: Marie Stopes and Annie Besant and Charles Bradlaugh in Britain, and Margaret Sanger in America. Women debilitated by the constant strain of pregnancy and childbirth no longer feature prominently in contemporary Britain, in which couples and individuals express expectations and plans of smaller and carefully spaced families. Yet it is not so long since large families were unavoidable and expected, sometimes consisting of fourteen or more live children, with the sorrowful experience of others who had died in infancy or childhood.

As a result of the publicity given to the early struggles for contraception and birth control, people's attitudes to family life and family size in the West began to change during the earlier part of this century. Vulcanized rubber, developed and produced during the 1930s, allowed refinements to be made to the male protective sheath, resulting in the rubberized condom. Letters desperately begging for advice were sent to the newly opened birth control clinics as people sought the information which they hoped would free them from 'the dread' of having to contemplate yet another child (original letters to Marie Stopes, M-O (Mass-Observation) Archive). The separation of men from their wives and families was a major factor in the fall in birth numbers throughout the Second World War and, despite the post-war baby boom, the birth rate never recovered to anything like its former state.

After the war ended, as well as people's relief and a sense of urgency towards the essential tasks of rebuilding the country and the economy, came an upsurge of people's confidence in the future and there was an awareness of, and an increase of interest in using, the contraceptive methods which were becoming more readily available. With the threat of war behind them people looked towards a more positive future and began to plan their lives with the realization that having children could be one part of the life of a married couple rather than the sole purpose of marriage. Cards of gratitude and letters of thanks were sent directly to Marie Stopes, portraying people's feelings of relief once they began to experience some measure of control in their reproductive lives (original letters, M-O Archive). Surveys conducted post-war by Mass-Observation showed that people had begun to consider and to state what they believed to be the right size for a family.

Reflections on their own birth-family lives, and the hardships endured by parents, particularly their mothers, stiffened people's resolve to ensure that their own, fewer, children would have a better life and that their own lives would not be so harsh. Whilst many respondents thought that 'no more than four' children was best, there were indications, even then, that others were already thinking around the replacement figure of only two and used 'one of each' to express their hopes and desires for a boy and a girl (original letters, M-O Archive). For the first time it became possible for people to have access to appropriate information and to feel confident that even such scant knowledge of preventative measures would enable them to exercise a measure of control over their reproductive lives in particular and their quality of life in general.

The opportunity of exerting some control over this vital aspect of life placed people in a position of being able to effect many changes: they began to question assumptions and go against traditions previously unchallenged or believed to be inevitable. A new generation of people were able to say, with the genuine authority and conviction of their own early life experiences, that giving birth to more children than could adequately be cared for and nurtured to healthy maturity, into families that were further impoverished by every new birth, was harmful for both parents and those children who were born. Theoretically, contraception was recognized as the means by which women might escape their destiny. At last it seemed that there was no longer any need to be a slave to biology (M-O Archive).

In the aftermath of the Second World War people mourned for the lives which had been lost but there was also a sense of recovery and hope for the future: an English future. The opening statement from a Mass-Observation publication spelled out its firm commitment to highlighting the dangers to the 'English race' of underpopulation.

The angle of approach is frankly partisan. Mass-Observation has lined up with those who do not want the English people to disappear . . . The plain and simple fact is that if eventually people do not decide to have more babies than they are having now, there will be no babies, no Englishmen or Englishwomen, for war or peace. (Mass-Observation, 1945, Preface)

This commitment had its roots firmly embedded in eugenics, a notion popularized in the early part of the twentieth century and made to appear reasonable by people in public life such as Havelock Ellis, H. G. Wells and George Bernard Shaw, as well as high-profile politicians, professionals and campaigners, including Dr Marie Carmichael Stopes who, above the many other birth control reformers of note in Britain and the parallel movements in America, stands out as being powerful in her advocacy, passionate in her beliefs and with a global influence which has carried through into contemporary life.

Marie Stopes was a believer in the ideals of married love and the joys of the marriage bed, and she wished for women to be relieved of the exhaustion of annual births and an inevitable increase in poverty in the lives of the working class. She was seemingly fearless in publishing and publicizing birth control information and providing practical help. Her desire was that women and men should have the opportunity to plan for fewer children and to enjoy those children who were born to them, but she was also a firm believer that the birth rate of the lower orders should not continue unchecked, subscribing to the eugenics creed of a 'weakening' of the race. She approved of the beliefs and aims of the Eugenics Society which had been founded in 1908 by Francis Galton, cousin to Charles Darwin, whose theory of natural selection was used to support the notion and possibility of using selective breeding to create human superiority.

A biography of Marie Stopes identifies the complexities of this extraordinary woman and the unnerving philosophy to which she subscribed. She is described as an elitist and an idealist, someone who envisaged a society made up of only the best and the beautiful if only the lower orders could be persuaded not to breed;

> She told the National Birth-Rate Commission, in her evidence in 1919, that the simplest way of dealing with chronic cases of inherent disease, drunkenness or bad character would be to sterilize the parents . . . To our ears, in the aftermath of Hitler, there is

something blood-chilling in her fearless quest for excellence, sacri-
ficing ordinary humanity on the altar of The Race. (Rose, 1992,
134)

Marie Stopes's pioneering spirit was only matched in America by Margaret Sanger who, in 1939, merged two of the organizations which she
had founded in order to create the single Birth Control Federation of
America, which later became the Planned Parenthood Federation of
America. A champion of women's reproductive rights and a forthright
and courageous birth control advocate, she also became the focus of
scandalized attention and was arrested on charges of obscenity in October 1916 for opening the Brownsville Clinic in Brooklyn, the nation's first
birth control clinic. As a nurse she had witnessed women suffering
through distressing and painful complicated births, seen the deprivation
and hardship caused to many people who had extremely large families,
and devoted her life to attempts to legalize birth control and the education of young women in order to lessen the incidence of unwanted
pregnancies and badly performed abortions. As well as educating women
and giving advice on family planning she provided any legal means of
birth control, also offering surgical procedures if necessary.

Despite their later falling-out, possibly because their single-mindedness
made them potential rivals (Rose, 1992), the depth of the commitment to
each other's work and the relationship which developed between the two
women is shown in Marie Stopes's campaigning to overturn the criminal
charges of illegal birth control propaganda brought by the US government against Margaret Sanger. Marie Stopes and other prominent people
wrote to President Wilson pleading that the charges of obscenity be
dropped 'in the interests of free speech and betterment of the race' (Rose,
1992). The petition gained wide publicity in Britain and sparked a similar
campaign in America, resulting in the case against Margaret Sanger being
dropped. The communications between the two women, as well as their
own prolific writings, make abundantly clear that there was a deep and
underlying passion and adherence to the notion of what both hailed as
'The Race'. Marie Stopes's immense influence on the birth control
movement in Britain is unchallenged and her initiatives in setting up
clinics and advice centres led to the global establishment of birth control
and reproductive health care advisory clinics (Leathard, 1980).

Contraception in contemporary contexts: post-war Britain and America

The assumption that all women want children and will strive to have them remained largely unchallenged throughout history (Firestone, 1970; Rowbotham, 1977; Rich, 1980; O'Brien, 1981 and 1989). The possibility that women could choose to remain without children has emerged as an issue and an area for discussion, debate and research only in recent years (Dowrick and Grundberg, 1980; Veevers, 1980; Campbell, 1985; Bartlett, 1994; Morell, 1994), and there has been an increasing dependence by women on new contraceptive methods, especially the oral contraceptive pill (Corea, 1985; Rowland, 1992; Hanmer, in Richardson and Robinson, 1993).

Without overmuch control from home, Church and state, a woman in the West need not reproduce year after year right through to the end of her reproductive life. Unlike other species who die soon after the completion of their biological breeding capacity, humans possess the potential for calculating and controlling their reproductive capability and a woman's life continues and is considered to be valuable and worthwhile for many years beyond her personal fertility timescale (Reed and Moriarty, 1980). Given good health and advantageous living conditions, women in the West may live for 40-plus years beyond menopause. If a woman had children in her twenties or thirties this may mean that for perhaps up to 50 years she is either controlling and regulating her reproductive system or continuing through life after the end of her fertility. For many women this phase of life is increasingly supported by hormone replacement treatment.

Throughout the 1970s and into the early 1980s the energy generated by second-wave feminism contributed to a developing positive atmosphere within which women could become more confident about the mechanics of their own bodies. Women's magazines picked up these issues and they became integrated into women's general understanding of aspects of their health and well-being. In this way many women gained a better understanding about how their bodies worked and such knowledge created opportunities for them to be interactive and assertive about medication, hospital treatment, medical advice and instructions, as well as becoming aware of the various debates about effective contraception and arguments about the hazards.

In Britain and in America many of the women's groups which existed at that time encouraged and made opportunities available for women to self-examine, a suggestion so wildly peculiar that the press made much of the experience and it became the target and substance of jokes and cartoons. Women exploring their own bodies and discovering their individual potential for sexual pleasure is frowned upon and heterosexual norms present the idea that satisfaction will be achieved only through penetrative sex, deemed to be the prerogative of the male. Even though a woman was not supposed to know about 'down there', that part of herself which would be for the pleasure of her husband or male partner, she was expected to be careful about its physical state, and even secretive about its natural, menstrual function.

> Part of the modesty about the female genitalia stems from actual distaste. The worst name anyone can be called is cunt. The best thing a cunt can be is small and unobtrusive: the anxiety about the bigness of the penis is only equalled by anxiety about the smallness of the cunt. No woman wants to find out that she has a twat like a horse-collar: she hopes she is not sloppy, or smelly, and obligingly obliterates all signs of her menstruation in the cause of public decency. (Greer, 1970, 39)

Through a learned ignorance, even fear and superstition about the mechanics of how their bodies worked, many women were vulnerable to the warnings and horror stories about pregnancy which, when mixed with the moral tales of not being 'an easy lay' may have had an effect on their potential for sexual expression and even their sexuality. Heterosexual women whose sexual lives started before the introduction of the oral contraceptive pill in the 1960s faced problems with assessing and making calculated judgements about what, for most women, was still the uncharted territory of their bodily rhythms. This was not only before it was introduced, but also before doctors were willing to prescribe the Pill to unmarried women, and well before the pregnancy advisory services were launched.

Women were cautious about paying the price of sexual pleasure through an unwanted pregnancy as well as ignorant about how to enjoy sex itself. As an illustration of this anxiety borne by many women during that time, Jean's diary noted that she had attended the local family planning clinic prior to her marriage and, after requesting information about contraception, she surprised the doctor by refusing an internal examination because she was still a virgin. She wrote, 'One reason for not having an active sex life then, of course, was the absolute dread of getting pregnant'.

Much second-wave feminist research focused on how women's oppression appeared to be inextricably bound up with motherhood yet, despite criticisms that motherhood is an oppressive state, becoming a mother remains a presumed and longed-for future for most women. Feminists writing in the 1960s and throughout the 1980s considered that women should seize whatever opportunities were offered to them, for example, the 'normal' female occupations within education or nursing, and then use such opportunities to define themselves within and carve a place beyond 'the patriarchal social relations in capitalist societies' (Hartmann, 1981). Many books of that era were written within the context of motherhood remaining an unquestioned future for women, although women were urged to seek for and develop a sense of self (Friedan, 1963). Hannah Gavron (1966) reported that, because of a post-war increase in the use of birth control methods, the women in her study could state with some confidence the number of children that they intended to go on to have, which was a measure of the speed with which many women took the opportunities offered by making use of birth control to plan the size of the family and to space the births of babies.

A major issue in many of the debates and disagreements surrounding women's control of their own fertility and their capacity to reproduce hinges on issues relating to women's choice and the potential for effective and active decision-making. Women, once in control of their own reproductive cycle are 'less dependent, more self-assured, more active. The spectre of independent women brings fear to the hearts of those who would maintain their power and privilege' (Huston, 1992). That spectre of independence may be the catalyst for an exercise of powers which effectively negates the choice and disempowers women's early struggles for greater autonomy and, whilst not necessarily making women into victims, the result of such power being exercised reminds women of the network of beliefs which reinforce expectations about how they should be. These social and cultural expectations and perceptions function as pressures which have a particular impact on women, thus narrowing and reducing opportunities for them to choose from wider life choices (Richardson, 1993).

The so-called sexual revolution which began in the early part of the

1960s had an irresistible effect on the old order. Many confrontations and battles around women's reproduction and the eventual passing of the 1967 Abortion Act increased the determination to fight to gain control over female bodies. There was heightened criticism of the repressive and punitive legislation which created obstacles to women having full and free access to contraceptive advice and facilities (regulations that they must be married, or showing evidence that they were engaged), as well as preventing women's access to safe abortion (illegal for all but health or psychological reasons). Pressure was increased from the action and political success of the National Abortion Campaign during the 1970s for women to be able to take control of their own fertility, for deciding when and how many children to have is vital for women to control this major aspect of their lives. However, 'the real barrier is men [as] children are often symbols of their maleness and virility' (*UN Chronicle*, September 1994).

Contemporary Western notions of sex are that it can be for either procreation or recreation, yet individuals often find themselves constrained by their own culture's understanding of what is considered to be appropriate sexual behaviour. As demonstrated by much historical evidence, the basis of many social and cultural standards suggested a conviction that it was normal and appropriate for women to be confined by 'Kirche, Küche, Kinder': Church, kitchen and children.

> men could assert their rights to a higher human and cultural life, women had to be satisfied with the narrow existence of kitchen, bedroom, and nursery, glorified as the happy home and family. In reality women were degraded to child raisers and domestic servants for men. To keep them in an inferior status, both church and state forbade them to make use of the available methods of birth control. 'Keep them barefoot and pregnant' is the most cynical expression of this male supremacy. Heaping insult on injury, women were then told they had been victimized not by class society but by nature, which decreed 'biology is woman's destiny'. (Reed and Moriarty, 1973, 4)

Although at a distance of two decades, the sentiments in this comment could still be applied to the lives of many women globally. Women face the often hazardous journey dictated by their bodies and must also gamble on being able to bring to bear some measure of control over their own reproduction, often within systems which appear to block their efforts to get information and advice, and seem intent on denying them access to contemporary contraceptive methods and birth control facilities.

Historically, there has been an increase of control by men over women's reproduction, with the elimination of women healers by a rising male-dominated medical profession (Ehrenreich and English, 1979; Taylor, 1996) which has encroached into women's control of birth. Recent archaeological research suggests that an ancient text, compiled by Hippocrates directly from oral traditions and containing detailed descriptions of female physiology, was most likely based on the knowledge of wise women and midwives. If this was the case, and he left unacknowledged the incorporation of their lore, such an act 'marks the earliest identifiable stage in the ongoing male takeover of the management of pregnancy and childbirth' (Taylor, 1996), and research in the area of medical sociology itself also is aware of and highly critical of what appears to be this 'takeover';

> In the case of human reproduction it is argued that greedy, selfish, and careless men expropriated from caring and careful midwives and lay women the power to help reproduce naturally, joyfully, and safely ... Gynaecology and family planning were similarly seen as having been taken over by medical men with questionable motives. (Porter, in Cunningham-Burley and McKeganey, 1990, 184)

Contemporary examples of such control over women's choices may be seen in the medicalization of pregnancy and also in the process of giving birth itself. Women birth attendants and midwives have been progressively demoted from the exclusively female process of birthing, allowing impersonal and rigid medical hierarchies to construct the type of regime (Hunt and Symonds, 1995) that women complain is like being treated like cows at a cattle market. Home births – much preferred by many women after experiencing the uncomplicated birth of the first child in hospital – continue to be unpopular with a male-medical model, as a birth which follows the natural rhythm of spontaneous birth is often inconvenient to the timetable and working patterns of hospital staff. Women given an expected date to give birth could find that, if labour did not begin spontaneously, they faced the intrusive and often painful process of being induced and, if there was a hint of trouble or potential

complications, they would find that they were to be prepared for Caesarian section regardless of their own wishes.

Dr Wendy Savage raised objections to what she saw as an alarming rise
in the incidence of Caesarian operations. She attempted to stand between
women's expressed preferences in their birth plans and views in the
medical world which ensured that women submitted to hospitalization
and labour ward regimes (Savage, 1986), yet she was immediately
suspended from a senior position and had to endure a personal and
vilifying attack which also impugned her professional competence. The
implication of this was likely to have been perceived as a loosening of the
complexity of professional controls over women's bodies which, in many
quarters of the medical establishment, continues to be thought of as
appropriate and proper but is subject to mounting criticism. Contemporary examples of research into the ways in which women are 'led into the
role of sick person' (Hunt and Symonds, 1995) also demonstrate that
many women find that the hospital experience is one which is highly
routinized by the birth attendants.

> Women who arrived at the labour ward were anxious, distressed,
> frequently observed to be in pain and generally unsure about what
> was to happen to them. They were subjected to a routine proce-
> dure which began with the removal of their clothes and ended with
> them being rendered powerless and attached to a fetal heart-rate
> monitor. (Hunt and Symonds, 1995, 74)

The extension of control over pregnancy and childbirth and now
conception itself has dangerous implications for women (Corea, 1985),
with coerced motherhood being the result of women having no right not
to reproduce (Rowland, 1992), and it is through heterosexuality and
marriage that men are accorded not only sexual access to women's bodies
but also have significant control over their reproduction (Brownmiller,
1975; Rowland, 1992). Social institutions, such as the family, reinforce
and maintain the patriarchal system and the controls embedded in law
and political systems and the diversity of religious beliefs and ideologies
contribute to the many ways in which women's access to contraception
and abortion are circumscribed, and also set the appropriate rates of
reproduction for women (Charles, 1993). Critics firmly assert (Overall, in
Overall, 1989) that a woman's body and her reproductive capacities
cannot be owned nor controlled by others, whether it be the foetus or its

father, her partner if she has one, and particularly not by doctors, the medical establishment or the state.

Contraception: global policy and government interests

> I believe that the NHS should provide sterilization on request – as with abortion – for women and men. It's an issue of reproductive rights which should have far more publicity. (Jill)

Contemporary battles over reproduction are fought on a global scale, in full public view, and in the contested arena of international conferences. Pro and anti population controllers and family planning representatives from governments, NGOs, women's rights organizations and those claiming religious interests construct local, national and international programmes for policy and action. Despite scare stories of food and fuel being depleted through overpopulation, population researchers are in general agreement that the causes of starvation, poverty and disease are determined by an unequal global distribution of food, medical supplies and care and not by shortages in world resources (Eversley and Kollmann, 1982; Findlay and Findlay, 1987; Goldscheider, 1992). They agree also that any solutions lie within the political arena rather than through even louder exhortations to limit family size and the supposedly unsustainable growth of world populations.

> At the core of the politics of birth control are issues of power and control. The power (or lack of power) occurs in two areas. One is in the development of contraceptives and the other is in access to existing birth control information and options. Technology and access determine the parameters of an individual woman's choice. (Colodny, in Overall, 1989, 30)

Whilst conferences and conventions are intended to have an effect on governments and policy-making, the outcome and undertakings for change as agreed by controllers, or in planning for the practical implementation of conference decisions, are made at levels above the lived experiences of most women. Once implemented, however, these agreements and changes in policy filter down, impinge upon and affect women's choices, decisions and action.

The population debate has moved on over the last twenty years, away from concentrating on the relationship between growth and economic development in the 1960s and 1970s and on to the current focus of sustainable development. This position acknowledges that diverse life-styles and contemporary human activity both affect and have damaging consequences for the ecological framework and hence for the capability of biological systems to meet the needs and demands placed on both renewable and non-renewable resources (Graham-Smith, 1994). This perspective has been reflected in world conferences (Johnson, 1994), most recently the 1994 Cairo International Conference on Population and Development, and the 1995 Beijing World Conference on Women.

The Cairo Conference, held over eleven days in September 1994, identified as a primary aim the stabilization of world population growth below the estimates of 7.5 billion, now predicted by 2015. One hundred and eighty countries with over two hundred speakers were represented at this fifth global concern conference[7] with many speakers emphasizing that population growth was not the only threat: destructive and unsustainable consumption patterns in the industrialized world would need to be acknowledged and steps taken to reduce their impact (from *UN Chronicle*, December 1994, 63–8). The majority consensus was that, through sustained economic growth and sustainable development, global population growth could be curbed over the next twenty years.

The tone of the conference was set by UN Secretary-General, Boutros-Ghali, who drew attention to the social and moral nature of the questions and issues to be considered, and reminded delegates that 'men and women throughout the world must have not only the right, but also the means to choose their families' futures'. The important role played by women in development was a permanent theme of the conference; Norway's Prime Minister, Gro Harlem Brundtland, spoke of the illusion of real development for many of the world's women, and she condemned the hypocrisy of a morality which may mean 'accepting mothers suffering or dying in connection with unwanted pregnancies and illegal abortions, and unwanted children living in misery' .

Many speakers also stressed the need for a holistic approach to concerns yet, even though the contribution of Pakistan's then Prime Minister Benazir Bhutto reflected this, she also emphasized that the conference outcome 'must not be viewed as a universal charter imposing sex education and abortion on individual cultures opposing such policies'. This was in contrast with (and appeared to challenge) the call from Boutros-Ghali for 'the right, and the means, to choose' for the individual.

The Vatican also made use of the conference to restate its position. In the preparatory stages the conference secretary Dr Nafis Sadik received a statement containing criticism from the Pope on potential decisions and measures which may undermine the family as being a 'natural, universal and fundamental institution, which cannot be manipulated without causing serious damage to the fabric and stability of society'. In this, the unchanging stance of Catholicism is reiterated:

> [the Church] stands opposed to the imposition of limits on family size, and to the promotion of methods of limiting births which separate the unitive and procreative dimensions of marital intercourse. Sterilization . . . because of its finality and its potential for the violation of human rights, especially of women, is clearly unacceptable . . . abortion, which destroys existing human life, is a heinous evil, and it is never an acceptable method of family planning. (In Johnson, 1994, 132)

This statement appears to demonstrate the total opposition of the Church to individuals using any planned method of contraception, much less interventionist approaches, which were the focus of much of the conference.[8] The Catholic Church confirmed its own part in opposing decisions that women may want to make about their own fertility and continues to condemn sterilization and abortion. In global terms these two methods, however unpalatable they may seem, appear to provide solutions for the inevitable consequences of lack of education, information and access to appropriate contraceptive methods. If available by choice, rather than coercion or force, both methods could offer opportunities to often desperate women and men for limiting family size and taking control of their own fertility.

The debates at Cairo about education programmes brought into sharp relief the use of birth control and medical intervention as important measures in controlling family size.[9] Neither abortion nor sterilization were seen as acceptable long-term solutions to limiting family size and controlling population growth, but speaker after speaker emphasized that programmes of family planning needed to include a full range of reproductive and primary healthcare services leading to fewer women seeking abortions. Overall, the focus which emerged stressed the need to harmonize population trends and patterns of development, thereby empowering women through genuine family planning choices and the control of their own fertility. Even set against what was reported as a 'backdrop streaked with controversy', the consensus was an acknowledgement that 'solutions to population problems must transcend mere demographics' with general agreement on the fundamental issue of transforming economically backward societies into modern ones. The closing chapters of the adopted programme emphasized the need for the provision of cost-effective educational programmes backed up by appropriate services and resources which would offer a wide range of options and would facilitate women's reproductive choices (*UN Chronicle*, December 1994).

Representative of the countries of the world were gathered at the 1995 Beijing 'World Conference on Women' with Baroness Chalker representing Britain. Her contribution concerned the ratification and implementation of all human rights conventions, especially those which relate to women and children, with an affirmation that the subjects addressed by the conference were not just 'women's issues'.

> Through women's lack of choice, patterns of gender inequality are perpetuated from one generation to the next. Progress for women is progress for all; families, the men, our children and our communities . . . If this Conference achieves only one thing it should be a global recognition of women's right to freedom of choice. (Baroness Chalker, Beijing, Sept. 1995; beijing-conf@tristram.edc.org)[10]

In her opening address to the conference, America's First Lady made clear her commitment to women's reproductive rights (and also, it would be fair to assume, that of the US government): in doing so she made a direct challenge to restrictions on and barriers to women's sexual and reproductive health:

> It is a violation of human rights when women are denied the right to plan their own families, and that includes being forced to have abortions or being sterilized against their will. If there is one message that echoes forth from this conference, it is that human rights are women's rights – and women's rights are human rights. (Hillary Rodham Clinton, Beijing, Sept. 1995; beijing-conf@tristram.edc.org)

Given the intervention of the Vatican at previous conferences where women's reproductive rights were debated, many delegates to the Beijing

Conference awaited the traditional papal condemnation of discussion and preparation for policy-making. However, apart from a rebuke at the preoccupation with sex and reproduction at the Conference, no bomb-shells were dropped. Instead what seemed to emerge was a softer, more tolerant line – but with a sting in the tail. Representing the Holy See and Pope John Paul II, Mary Ann Glendon reminded the conference of the Pope's *Letter to Women* in which he acknowledged the deficiencies of past positions, including those of the Catholic Church, and made reference to the historical oppression of women. She said that the Holy See welcomed the aim of freeing women from the unfair burdens of cultural conditioning as their dignity and rights are essential for the construction of a stable society. If women are to enjoy their rights, however, their roles within the family must not be undermined, as 'these roles are inseparably linked to their commitments to God, family, neighbour and especially their children'. Using the term 'feminization of poverty', the Pope urged governments and husbands (though not women themselves) to strive to address those social factors which oppress women and to seek to provide opportunities for advancement so as to lessen the burden on working mothers and sole providers for families.

Mary Ann Glendon asserted that it was a travesty to say that the Catholic Church's teaching supported procreation at all costs, but it did condemn coercion in population policies and possible health risks associated with family planning methods, especially experimental ones. She said that the conference did not place sufficient emphasis on widespread sexual permissiveness and the consequent threat to women's health, and that abortion should not be promoted as a means of family planning, but that efforts should be made to eliminate factors which lead women to seek abortions. A woman or girl who is pregnant, frightened and alone must be offered a better alternative than the destruction of her unborn child (taken from 'Vatican raps women's meeting', 26 Sept. 1995; beijing-conf@tristram.edc.org).

The adopted programmes of the conferences emphasized the urgent need to produce and make provision for contraceptive commodities and services of high quality supported by appropriate information and education to be delivered in a socially responsible, culturally sensitive, acceptable and cost-effective manner. By making available birth control and contraceptive resources and facilities, and without either pressure or coercion, the option to use them at least allows women the opportunity to take greater care of their own health. This then may prove useful as a factor which stabilizes the family unit and its economy, within which so many women and their children live.[11]

> The prevailing gap between women's ideal family size and actual childbearing suggests that women's reproductive aspirations are seldom fulfilled. The inadequate control women have over their reproduction is also evident from the high prevalence of unplanned childbearing. (taken from WOM/866 15 Sept. 1995; beijing-conf@tristram.edc.org)

The ethical context within which current debates rage about contraception is one which acknowledges that prohibitions on birth control have been a feature of many past societies and cultures as much for reasons considered socially necessary (post-war, for example) as for those spiritual and moral (Fromer, 1983). Contemporary ethical issues are of a global nature, with the distribution and use of world resources, national public policies and money for population control programmes, presenting as highly contentious because of their perceived potential relationship with racist or discriminatory policies. Coerced and forced sterilization are examples of a paternalistic interference by the state into the individual's reproductive privacy (Fromer, 1983) and have social, cultural, psychological and racial overtones (Greer, 1984; Humm, 1989).

If allowed access to the wide range of contraceptive and post-conception methods, and given essential information about their own fertility, women believe themselves to be better placed – and infinitely better able than men – to make judgements about their bodies and lives. In all of the debates about contraception and abortion, whether medical, social or moral, what must be borne in mind is that, regardless of the attitudes and legislation of any society, individual women will carry on doing what women have done for thousands of years; that is, seeking to prevent conception, aborting an unwanted foetus or abandoning or killing a newborn child.

Contemporary developments in contraception

In 1984, Germaine Greer's work, *Sex and Destiny*, was subject to widespread disapproval and condemnation from some feminists and sections of the media because she appeared to be calling for an approach to sex which bordered on a return to the chastity belt or, at the very least, self-discipline and periods of abstinence from heterosexual activity. The chapter which appeared to create such a furore ('Chastity is a form of birth control'), which read as a critical as well as a polemic piece of writing, deserved more than just dismissal. Eleven years on, and probably not for the same reasons that Greer propounded, women were reporting making not only a childfree choice but also a sexfree choice.

The findings of the 1995 General Household Survey on contraceptive use pointed towards 40 per cent of single women (never married and not cohabiting), aged 16 to 49, saying that they did not use contraception because they were not having sex. The percentage of women who were defined as widows, divorcees or separated and who said that they were not in a sexual relationship was 34 per cent; there was even a zero sex rating for 1 per cent of married women or women living with a male partner. As with so many findings, it is vital to take into account what was unasked or left unsaid, for example the numbers of sexually active lesbian women not in heterosexual relationships and so presumably not needing to use contraception who may have responded, and of the women who were unwillingly celibate.

Celibacy and abstinence aside, there remains an essential post-AIDS need for increased safety and security in the choice and availability of barrier and other contraceptive methods. Continuing research has created even more diversity, and the FPA defines the methods currently in use worldwide as: combined and progesterone-only oral contraceptive pill; male and female condoms; diaphragm; cap; injectables; implants (e.g. Norplant); natural family planning (including the latest, Persona); intrauterine devices (e.g. Copper 7), intrauterine system (IUD plus slow hormone release); female sterilization; and male vasectomy. Experiments with a male contraceptive pill are ongoing but its initial reception by potential male-users was not encouraging:

> There is a trial underway (Edinburgh Royal Infirmary) for the male pill which contains a synthetic version of progesterone. The brain sends messages to the testes to stop producing testosterone and sperm and an implant or six-monthly injection counteracts this loss of testosterone. According to the coordinator of the research team there will be side effects and most men will not relish having to endure regular injections. The necessarily higher dose of

testosterone in a further pill can have an effect on the liver and the blood. (*Guardian*, 18 March 1997)

Of the other new product developments (all for women) some are already showing signs of problems in use. Persona, one of the so-called 'natural' methods, is regarded with some scepticism by the Family Planning Association, and family planning advisers consider it to be a fertility monitor and not a contraceptive. With a projected 5 per cent failure rate, considerably higher than condom use, Marie Stopes's clinics are having to deal with Persona's initial failures, and for women not in permanent or established relationships, or who have sex at unpredictable intervals, natural methods are likely to present the greatest hazard to becoming pregnant.

Norplant is a method which involves inserting under the skin (probably of the upper arm) six matchstick-sized 'rods' containing a progesterone hormone. This can be performed under local anaesthetic, in the GP's surgery or a family planning clinic, taking approximately twenty minutes, and giving up to five years' protection against pregnancy. In the four years after its launch in Britain in 1993 and two years after its first use in America, 52,000 women chose Norplant. The main reason is likely to be that it need not be monitored and continues to be effective throughout that time which is, of course, also a disadvantage. Currently (1997) there is no national register of Norplant users nor are women yet on a central register acting to issue reminders to renew or replace the contraceptive; without this, woman may be at risk of becoming pregnant.

A major difficulty is that there is a tendency for the rods to be difficult to be removed, particularly if they have not been inserted by a trained practitioner. As with many of the new technologies, this method also is not without its own early problems:

> All [she] wanted was not to have any more children. A mother-of-two she thought the new contraceptive implant, Norplant, would end her worries about pregnancy. Instead [she] has endured two and a half years of ill health, pain and worry. The stress has been so great for her and her family that it nearly destroyed her marriage. Today, she and her husband are back together, but she cannot forget Norplant and its legacy. (*Birmingham Evening Mail*, 23 Jan. 1997)

The problem for this woman, and others who have reported severe side effects and reactions and have attempted to have Norplant removed, is that she has had to endure operations (two, so far, under general anaesthetic) to extract one of the rods which is too close to a nerve in her arm to be removed without damage. Apart from the pains and restricted movement in her arm, she has also found that the word most appropriate to describe her menstruation was 'haemorrhage'.[12] The manufacturers of Norplant in expressing their own concerns are supported by leading specialists and family planning advisers, who point out that, of the now 42,000 users in the country, only a very small number have been disadvantaged, although the stories from those few who do experience problems with this and other chemical-based contraceptives are given high-profile reporting: this is reflected in the misgivings some women have about putting chemicals into their bodies over a number of years of their fertile lives.[13]

Cost may be a factor in women receiving whichever contraceptive method is deemed to match their needs, as GPs are now conscious of having to work within budgets. Mirena is an intrauterine system combining the effects of a coil and an implant with controlled hormone release over three years. It has been shown to be highly reliable in trials but because, at £100, it costs ten times more than the fitting of standard IUDs, it is extremely costly for women to have it fitted. Family planning doctors, however, give it high praise, saying that Mirena is the most significant advance in reversible contraception since the invention of the pill. There are many reports of additional bonuses in the use of Mirena, such as in controlling heavy and painful bleeding and a very low incidence of ectopic pregnancy. Nevertheless, for women who are cautious about long-term effects on their body, Mirena is yet another chemical and unsuitable for childfree women who are not seeking to use reversible contraceptive methods.

> the contraceptive services currently available to women in Britain fall a long way short of meeting women's own contraceptive needs and desires . . . current developments in the marketing and targeting of implantable hormonal contraceptives should leave women in little doubt that the health care industry intends to continue its control over their fertility . . . women's own needs [take] a rather poor second place to the interests of contraceptive manufacturers,

the medical profession, the government, and ultimately all sexually active heterosexual men. (Foster, 1995, 28)

Contraception in Britain

Despite an assumption of its almost universal use, the Pill is not suitable for all women. Other methods, with their much higher failure rate, may cause the type of scare which could be the catalyst for a woman's determination to put an end to monthly methods with the bonus of security and peace of mind brought about by sterilization. There is likely to have been a discussion about who will be the one to be sterilized within a permanent relationship (Allen, 1985; Bartlett, 1994; Family Planning Association, *passim*), with the option of male vasectomy also a possibility. The women in this study, however, were very clear that the decision for sterilization as a final method of contraception was their own.

The UK General Household Survey of 1995 identified that contraception for women aged between 16 and 49 years was divided into categories, of which the safe period, cap, withdrawal and IUD were shown as being least popular, and with condoms (18 per cent) and the Pill (25 per cent) accounting together for almost half of the methods used. Whilst the proportion of all women using the Pill rose slightly, from 22 per cent in 1989 to 23 per cent in 1993, it has stayed constant at 25 per cent since then. The percentage of women using the Pill in the 35 to 39 years age bracket, however, has risen 12 per cent in nine years, up from 8 per cent in 1986 to 20 per cent in 1995. In part this is because of the ubiquitous place of the Pill in contemporary Western society and also because there have been significant changes and reported 'improvements' in the various chemical constituents of the many brands of pill (such as the progesterone-only mini pill), resulting in GPs and contraceptive-advice services being in a position to recommend and prescribe what they believe to be the most appropriate pill for individual needs.

The surprising finding from the 1995 study is that the figure for sterilization is 24 per cent. Although this includes both male and female surgical procedures, 5 per cent of women under 30 have been sterilized.[14] As well as a very small number of childfree women electing to be sterilized, the majority of women who opt for sterilization believe that they have completed their families. Other women who make up the figure of 24 per cent will be those who have had serious medical reasons for sterilization, hysterectomy for ovarian or other cancers, or in an attempt to curtail chronic and debilitating conditions, such as hysterectomy for fibroids or excessively difficult or painful menstruation (dysmenorrhoea), or essential emergency operations after ectopic pregnancy or a clumsy attempt at abortion. There will also be a smaller number who are sterilized for what may be euphemistically termed 'social reasons'.

> There will be a significant number of other women who have never been pregnant who are sterilized, such as the handicapped, and the Down's Syndrome. These girls can't have ordinary contraceptives – like IUDs or Norplant – it's decided by advisers, her social workers, and the parents. It's easier to give an anaesthetic and sterilize her, but it's not her choice, it's because the family say they can't bring up children. (family planning nurse)[15]

A number of scares have erupted in recent years over the potential long-term dangers which accompany Pill use and these are often the signal for many women immediately to stop using the Pill until fears are calmed, although some may never return to it as a method. Unwanted conceptions and pregnancies are the unfortunate and traumatic result of oral contraceptives being identified by name (publicity in 1995 named a number of the 'mini pills'), and there is a predictable rise in abortions in the aftermath of such publicity:

> In the year following the 1995 scare, there were 94,160 fewer prescriptions for the Pill, normally prescribed to three million women, and a 6 per cent rise in unwanted pregnancies. ('Avoiding the bitter morning-after pill', *Guardian*, 18 March 1997)

Annual holidays and festivities are also a major cause of fears of unwanted pregnancy. Many women no longer wait for confirmation of pregnancy and instead seek immediate intervention, 'just in case'. A method growing in popularity and used more and more as an emergency measure is the 'morning-after' pill. A regional newspaper report highlighted this:

> Counsellors at Birmingham family planning clinics have been flooded with SOS calls from worried women seeking emergency contraception. Demand soared in the days leading up to Christmas (of 1996) when clinics were inundated with people seeking

advice after office parties . . . requests have continued to climb as clients count the costs of their festive flings. ('Scramble for the morning-after pill', *Birmingham Evening Mail*, 2 Jan. 1997)

If all else fails, women in the developed world have the opportunity of applying for termination of pregnancy. This remains an area of difficulty for many women, who have to deal not only with the practical aspects and physical trauma pre and post operation but also with emotional stress and any struggle with personal conviction or misgivings. Women for whom pregnancy and motherhood is not questioned may also find themselves compromised by an unexpected conception and there is a suggestion that mistakes and what women describe as 'getting caught' account for many babies, unplanned but usually welcomed, at least outwardly. As well as facing social disapproval, women who do not want to have children may struggle silently with personal uncertainties for some time. They are keenly aware of the presentation of motherhood as being normal and expected of them and Linda L. believes 'it's your own self-will against the media and all the messages you get. It's such hard work having children and I believe there's many women who don't want them.' Those working with birth control and women's fertility are aware of a woman's ambivalence in being pregnant by accident and only later, as a consequence of that, coming to want the baby.

> I think most women can't say why they just know they don't want children – but that's the same even for women with children! Am I cynical? The reason women have children is by accident, often failed contraception, then they have a pregnancy test, and I say 'How do you feel about that, are you happy?' and they say to themselves 'Oh well, will it make any difference . . .? Oh, I suppose it's alright . . .' Even if they hide it for a while as soon as people know, the woman has to be pleased and if she's not thrilled to bits and if she wants a termination – well, the guilt is there, immediately. (family planning nurse)

Condemnation of abortion and physical attacks on abortion clinic personnel are on the increase and anti-abortion groups showed a high profile in the run-up to the 1997 General Election. Up to 50 MPs who support women's rights to abortion were targeted for criticism and censure and prominent Church leaders attacked the (then) Opposition

Leader, Tony Blair, accusing him of 'washing his hands' of the issue because he had never voted against abortion in any of the votes in the House of Commons. Cardinal Basil Hume, the head of the Roman Catholic Church in England and Wales, accused Tony Blair and others of 'fudging the issue by pretending that they held a quasi pro-life position', and Hume gained great publicity in his campaign to make abortion a major issue in the election. His main message to all anti-abortion supporters and activists spoke of 'the great evil in our society which is unworthy of a civilised society', and in his later interview with GMTV's Sunday programme he reiterated that the Roman Catholic Church would never change its attitude towards abortion.[16] Even after the election, Hume continued his attack on Labour Party policy preparations for government, demanding that Tony Blair 'take a stand' against abortion (Radio 4 *News*, Sunday 5 May 1997).

None of the childfree women in this study saw abortion as an easy birth control option and most were definite that part of their decision to apply for sterilization was to avoid having to consider abortion. The often lengthy delays and more often outright refusals of their applications from GPs and consultants increased their anxiety and inhibited their potential for relaxed, enjoyable heterosexual activity, free from the fear of an unwanted pregnancy.

Sterilization as a birth control option

The incidence of sterilization has shown a dramatic leap, from 4 per cent in 1970 to its high of 24 per cent in 1995, and it is likely that the reasons for this lie in the interrelationship between the medical and social arenas. As the techniques for the operation developed and made surgery simpler and less intrusive (hence less hazardous), and with the family complete, individuals began to consider male and female sterilization as one of many contraceptive alternatives. Thus, sterilization has extended and broadened the horizons of birth control measures, yet, as a surgical procedure, it is not without hazards. There is a greater risk of ectopic pregnancy in sterilized women because, as they continue to ovulate, there remains the slight (but potentially life-threatening) chance of fertilization in the fallopian tube. Depending on the method used, and with a failure rate of one to three in one thousand, it is the safest method of all contraception, bar celibacy. Even so, women do still become pregnant.

A Birmingham woman has become pregnant in a million to one chance after being sterilized. Mother-of-four Mrs R. aged 25 said she would keep the baby but would sue (a hospital in Birmingham) over the error. She decided on the sterilization when it became clear that her youngest child of 14 months was handicapped and required extra care. 'I was sterilized in May and was nine weeks pregnant and had the child aborted. I went through hell afterwards, and I can't go through that again, so I will have the child.' (It was reported that a 'clamp' on the fallopian tube had become dislodged.) (*Birmingham Evening Mail*, 28 Dec. 1996)

Nevertheless, despite the rise in popularity of sterilization with women and men, it is becoming increasingly difficult to obtain NHS referral and more and more people are resorting to private clinics and hospitals. However difficult this may be for those who seek sterilization in order to prevent further births, the refusal rate is inevitably greater for those who apply with the intention of preventing any births at all. The first to suffer from cutbacks in these services are childfree women, so that a woman who had no children would be seen as not having priority for sterilization whereas, for example, a woman with eight children would be viewed more sympathetically (Grigg, in Bartlett, 1994).

Jane Bartlett interviewed fifty-plus childfree women, including eleven who had been sterilized (Bartlett, 1994) and suggests a national figure of approximately 3 per cent of sterilized women who are childfree compared with 45 per cent of sterilized women who have had three or more children. Because many of that 3 per cent may include women who are sterilized for reasons such as those already explored (e.g. gynaecological or other medical reasons, or 'social reasons'), it is much more likely that elective sterilization by childfree women for contraceptive reasons is an even smaller figure, possibly statistically almost unrecordable. None of the medics other than Professor Winston could do other than give a 'guesstimate' (and even he was cautious about precise figures) and most suggested that there is currently no data available which would be accessible for research:

There are very few women about who have been sterilized with no children. I may have seen one or two but it's very uncommon. Almost all the figures will relate to people who have completed their families. Nulliparous women, the women who have never borne children, who are sterilized I would think would be less than half than one per cent of the figures. You won't find separate figures – and also you won't have information on who later regretted it . . . (Consultant A.)

As well as the lack of such a breakdown of existing available medical information and data which would allow an examination of the numbers of childfree women who elect to be sterilized, there is also no way of identifying how many women apply to GPs but are not referred on. This may be because of their reluctance in referring an otherwise healthy woman for a procedure of this type (particularly if they are under the age of 30) or an awareness on the part of the GP that such an application has little chance of immediate success. Yet a number of studies, including this one, identify that women who have decided to remain childfree and are resolute and determined to pursue sterilization continue to apply and reapply for the operation despite social condemnation and a medical profession which refuses to consider that they could make such a serious decision about their reproductive lives (Newton, 1984; Bartlett, 1994).

Such dismissive attitudes raised fury in the responses of the diarists in this study. They emphasized that the permanence of sterilization had been impressed upon them and that the operation must be considered to be non-reversible, but that no such warnings appear to be given to women considering motherhood, even though after childbirth there is little chance of a return to a childfree lifestyle.[17] The diaries and interviews were full of exasperation at what the diarists perceived as a glaring anomaly, which they felt may have had a bearing on the way they were treated by society in general and the medical profession in particular. Vicky's decision not to have a child drew attention to the absence of any understanding about such a choice: 'it's like you can have children willy-nilly all over the place but you can't possibly make the opposite decision', and Helen made a point which, in a variety of ways, was a theme in the diaries and during the interviews:

I think that if a woman of 16 is able to decide to have a baby then a woman of the same age should be able to decide not to. After all both decisions are irreversible and it's easier to adopt, or to foster, or to have IVF if there's a change of mind, than it is to pass a child over to Social Services if you have a change of mind about that . . . (Helen)

Yet this appears to be a further way of women dividing against each other. If the outcome of opting for sterilization is for a childfree woman never to have any children, and for a woman with children not to have any more, then it appears to be the decisions made by medical gatekeepers which create tensions between women and not the decisions of the women themselves. The anger and fury expressed by childfree women, who are sure that they will not change their minds after sterilization, towards women who have been sterilized after completing their families and who later change their minds, may be seen as misdirected. It is doctors and consultants who make decisions about sterilization, based on available information which informs them that a significant number of women who opt for this procedure do, indeed, later have regrets and return requesting reversal. However, this number is likely to be over-whelmingly made up of women who have had children and opted for sterilization so as to have no more.

Because childfree women electing for sterilization is an unresearched area and the number of women involved is small, medical staff use the studies and research currently relevant to reach what seems to them to be appropriate conclusions. Much of their consideration is based on an undeniable awareness that, however determined a woman is, and how-ever firm her decision not to have any children or any more children, ongoing life experiences may affect that choice; for example, an unplan-ned pregnancy often does result in an acceptance and welcoming of motherhood, or changed circumstances such as a new relationship may generate maternal feelings. In such instances, and far from a changed choice being fickle or evidence of their capricious nature (occasionally voiced during interviews with medical practitioners), these women may reverse or adapt and adjust any previously made decisions which they decide are outdated and no longer appropriate in their lives. None the less, this study asserts that there does seem to be an identifiable difference between women who have become mothers, and women who say that they had 'always known' that they wanted to remain without children, and this difference must necessarily be part of future thinking around any medical decision on any application for sterilization from a childfree woman.

As a major social institution which profoundly affects all individuals, medicine and the medical profession have been widely criticized, espe-cially by birth control campaigners and by feminists, for preventing women from managing their own bodies and controlling their own fertility. Even while doctors in the West appear to be reluctant to agree to the elective sterilization of childfree women, as they believe there is a high possibility of later regrets and requests for reversal, conversely there is increased interest and involvement (as well as much social and medical sympathy and support for couples) in the reproductive technologies for infertility. Currently, there seems to be an absence of any question about whether or not these potential parents may regret having the child that they so desperately desire. This anomalous attitude attracts the criticism that doctors seek to maintain control not only over those whom they decide to assist to have children but also, because of their reluctance to take childfree women seriously then refusing their applications for sterilization, that they continue to exert their power over those whom they decide they will not help.

Notes

1. John Vidal's summary of three reports: the Panel on Sustainable Development, British Government; the Worldwatch Institute, Washington; the United Nations Environment Agency, Nairobi (*Guardian*, 28 Jan. 1997, p. 4).
2. *Sunday Pictorial* headlines, 1949, source Mass-Observation Archive, University of Sussex in Brighton.
3. A fall or rise in the rates of birth does not occur by chance nor simply as a result of the private decisions and actions of individuals. Government policy-making, as much as anything else, is a powerful dynamic behind the figures and reports of enforced childbearing in Romania and the single child policy in China provide contemporary examples of this. Globally, sterilization is the most used method of birth control, although it is reported as being part of population control programmes which include compulsion and coercion. During the 1995 Beijing World Conference on Women there was a stream of information on the Internet, including the following from official websites (September 1995):

   The Chairman of an American Congressional Delegation, attending the United Nations Women's Conference in Beijing, sharply criticized China for human rights abuses . . . Congressman Christopher Smith was especially scathing in his criticism of what he said was a Chinese practice of forced abortion and sterilization to carry out its 'one-child-per-family' policy. He said that Chinese denials, that forced abortion and sterilization are official, are nonsense. (Websites: beijing conf@tristram.edc.org/ beijing95-l@netcom.com September 1995)

4. It was interesting to note that the Mass-Observation publication *Britain and Her Birth-Rate* set out what appears to be a 'Malthus in reverse' notion of an annual population decrease of 3 per cent in Britain. The projection was that by the year

2015 the population would be 10,456,000 which would be made up of 3 per cent in the age range 0–14, 44 per cent of 15–59, and 53 per cent of 60-plus.

5. The book had what was considered to be the shameless subtitle, 'How a woman should order herself during pregnancy, in the lying-in room, and after delivery, with hints on the management of the baby, and on other matters of importance, necessary to be known by married women'.

6. Early birth control history is thoroughly researched and well documented elsewhere.

7. Previous conferences on population and development were held in Rome in 1954, Belgrade in 1965, Bucharest in 1974 and in Mexico City in 1984.

8. Even if she had no short-term effect on the Catholic Church, Marie Stopes was very influential in the changes made to the thinking of other religious leaders. In her conclusion to the biography of Marie Stopes, June Rose writes, 'if she had tilted at windmills she had also slain giants. In July 1958, almost forty years after Marie had first revealed her "message" to the Anglican Bishops at the Lambeth Conference, the Conference acknowledged the necessity for birth control and vindicated Marie Stopes's "obscene" ideas in words that might have been dictated by Marie herself. "The procreation of children is not the sole purpose of Christian marriage; implicit within the bond of husband and wife is the relationship of love with its sacramental expression in physical union . . . the responsibility for deciding upon the number and frequency of children has been laid by God upon the conscience of parents everywhere".' (in Rose, 1992, 244–5).

9. For example, studies show estimates that in Chile in 1993 'nearly one third of the women who controlled their fertility had undergone this treatment (sterilisation)' (Johnson, 1994). Similarly, in the USA, figures show that the sterilization rate among Black peoples is 45 per cent higher than among whites, with as many as 42 per cent of all American Indian women and 35 per cent of Puerto Rican women having been sterilized.

10. The full reference is: Baroness Chalker of Wallasey, Minister of State for Foreign and Commonwealth Affairs and Minister for Overseas Development of the United Kingdom, Beijing, Sept. 1995 (beijing-conf@tristram.edc.org)

11. Both conferences, focusing on women's lives and based on the premiss of population and birth control, considered only heterosexual attitudes and activity, and family life as being normal. With biology used to explain the social differences between women and men, women's reproductive capacity served to justify the gendered perspective that all women are naturally heterosexual (Stacey, in Richardson and Robinson, 1993). Because of this, an issue of major importance to feminists and relevant to debate was ignored or given no credibility: that is, the criticism that heterosexuality is compulsory and an institution which suppresses and denies other sexualities.

12. Other women also report what they describe as heavy bleeding, excessive weight gain and bloating and all of the symptoms which most women would recognize as that catch-all phrase, premenstrual tension or syndrome. This seems often to be used nowadays as a term which describes anything from feelings of mild irritation to rushes of murderous rage.

13. Several diarists wrote or spoke about this worrying aspect of taking the Pill, with Linda L. commenting that she often wondered just what ten years of taking chemicals had done to her; her response was to stop taking it.

14. This appears to be an extraordinarily high percentage given the hostility reported

towards them by the women in this study. Currently, there are no nationally available collated figures to consider and analyse the breakdown of women into categories such as 'childfree elective', 'with children elective', 'childfree non-elective', etc.

15. During 1997 there were 'shock-horror' reports of the discovery that Sweden had operated a system of enforced sterilization upon certain types of people in the population. Despite the often offhand comments and even direct references, such as the one given here to me, as yet there is no similar uproar against this type of operation, for 'social reasons', being carried out in Britain despite its potential link with eugenics.

16. There were many media reports on this at the time. The extracts from the Cairo and Beijing conferences in this chapter may also throw light on this attitude.

17. Some diarists made dry asides to the effect that it appears that only as part of the rigorous screening for adoption is there ever any suggestion that there could be a factor called 'suitable' when it comes to parenting. I also came across medical references on the types of women who may be considered 'suitable' for sterilization which appeared to be based mainly on consultants' subjective opinions about the woman's level of intelligence, or signs of fecklessness or absence of morals (from personal interviews, and in Allen, 1985).

3

Examining the Childfree Choice: From Contraception to Sterilization

My decision to be sterilized triggered off a huge mix of responses in others. One close friend was angry and said that R. should have a vasectomy but others were incredibly shocked that I was making the decision irrespective of him. The worst responses were from those with no kids and one who couldn't have any said it felt like I was kicking her in the teeth. This was so offensive as I'd been really supportive to her. Another who was pregnant felt it was a criticism of her choice, but one friend who'd become a mother was angry in a different way, she said 'God, I've really fallen for it, why didn't I see it?'. It's the doing that's deeply threatening. If you're not sterilized, the blow is softened – there's still a chance and they say, 'Well, she might still have a baby . . .'. (Jude)

Many assumptions about childfree motivations were voiced again and again during the course of the research and, like much conjecture, were seldom borne out. One opinion that frequently occurred was that women who choose not to have children are themselves 'loners', probably isolates and with no brothers or sisters, but of the 23 women in the study only four mentioned being an only child. There also seemed to be a view that women without children must dislike them yet, although 'I never wanted children' was a common statement in the diaries, only three women said specifically that they did not like children, and most others said that they 'weren't interested' or 'had no interest' in children. Most of the women were keenly aware of the impact on their lives of an unknown newcomer and Vicky expressed her puzzlement at the eagerness of potential parents to 'invite a stranger into their life and relationship', adding 'after all, you don't know who or what you are getting'.[1]

A further assumption was that women would only need to have the experience of conceiving or of being pregnant and that, in itself, would bring about a rush of maternal instinct, but the fear of an unwanted pregnancy was a constant theme throughout the diaries and during the interviews. Eight women had experienced pregnancy and a further one had carried the baby to full term then given up the baby for adoption. Of these, two women said that they had had early miscarriages and five had opted for termination of the pregnancy, with one woman undergoing the distress of four abortions: these were as a result of contraceptive failure on each occasion and before she could convince a consultant to take seriously her request for sterilization.

On a few occasions during interviews with medical staff, the view was expressed that many determinedly childfree women become pregnant by accident, go on to have the baby and then find the mothering experience fulfilling and worthwhile, and so were clearly wrong in their earlier decision to remain childfree. This seems to ignore that there is a profound difference between a childfree woman and a woman who is pregnant. Once pregnant, a woman faces a very different set of issues from those she would use in asserting and maintaining her childfree state. Being childfree and stating the intention to remain so is of a different order from being pregnant and making the same statement. To remain childfree when not pregnant entails a woman maintaining her vigilance about effective contraception and that, necessarily, includes access to abortion without which she cannot be in total control of her own fertility (Jacobson, 1990).

Given the difficulties reported by most of the women with method contraception and taking account of the incidental and informal references to problems when women talk together, it does not seem surprising that women terminate a pregnancy if, despite their best efforts or if they have unprotected sex, they find themselves pregnant. Jill had had a scare and knew what her reaction would have been if the test had been positive: 'When I was two weeks late I was shit-scared and there was no doubt about it. I thought, of course I'll have an abortion.' Jude lived in a state of permanent fear of pregnancy prior to her sterilization:

> I hated taking the Pill and would take occasional 6-month breaks where we would use condoms or just not have vaginal penetrative sex. A couple of times I forgot the Pill so, on two occasions, I had to take the 'morning-after' pill. We regularly had scares and if I ever thought I was pregnant (which was every other month!) I would be terrified and have always been very clear that I would have a termination. There was always a pregnancy testing kit in the bathroom and I would have considered abortion, if it had become necessary. Fortunately, I have never had to do that. (Jude)

The majority of the women in this study made it clear that, if necessary, they would not have hesitated to arrange for termination of an unplanned pregnancy. As well as the women who had been pregnant and had had terminations, miscarriages or (in one case) gave birth followed by the adoption of the baby, a further four women stated quite clearly that they would have sought abortion had the scares been early pregnancies. Jean, however, was definite that she would not have done so:

> I'd been taking the Pill even after getting a divorce – just in case. I did wonder at one point and that was scary but the test came back negative. I would not have had an abortion. I suppose there are religious reasons for me, but I'm not anti-abortion. I'm sure that I would have considered adoption – even if I wouldn't have gone through with it. (Jean)

Many women do resort to abortion if there has been a failure of contraception or if they are unwillingly pregnant, even if they have already had children or intend to do so in their future. The diarists' stories confirmed and emphasized that, in order to retain her childfree state, a pregnant woman must consider and take the traumatic but necessary action to terminate a pregnancy, the only decision which will allow her to return to being childfree.

The process of consideration of personal issues and the decision to undergo abortion is one which many women face. Pauline's story was additionally complex in that she was facing not only an unplanned pregnancy, but also the possibility of the death of her second husband.

> I used a pregnancy-testing kit and was in a state of horror and absolute disbelief when it registered positive . . . because earlier that year my husband had been diagnosed with cancer . . . We had long discussions about what to do . . . I wondered whether it was my destiny to have a child who would be something to remember my husband by or – because of his illness – I might be left nursing a sick husband and a child, like a single mother with very little financial support. My answer came when I was sitting in my GP's reception area, urine sample in hand, surrounded by women in various states of pregnancy. I suddenly got a very clear sense of being in the wrong place and asked myself what was I doing there . . . I had a strong sense of panic. Even then, I might have gone through with it, who knows? In the event I miscarried at ten weeks. (Pauline)

Resorting to abortion is likely to be viewed with as much distaste by childfree women as it is by many other women, and there is little evidence and only anecdote to support the pervasive charge that there are large numbers of women who use abortion as contraception. Women's language is peppered with references to children whose births are described as 'mistakes' or 'unplanned' but whose arrival was accommodated and accepted as inconvenient, rather than rejected and dealt with as unacceptable. It may be that women who are determined to remain childfree are more likely to seek abortion immediately they conceive than do women who see motherhood and children as part of their future lives.

Most women who have decided against having children are loath to take the final step which ends their fertility even if they are prepared to go through with abortions or morning-after precautions. By remaining notionally fertile, they feel that they continue to have a stake in the future (Greer, 1984) and this is confirmed in many of the previous studies of childfree women who continue to use contraception and who, if they had considered it at all, rejected sterilization. The majority feeling from the childfree women in Jane Bartlett's study (Bartlett, 1994) is that the finality of such an action would be too permanent and they voiced concerns which were not necessarily about becoming mothers but were about keeping the choice open because, for them, 'it's damn difficult to slam that door shut once and for all' (Morell, 1994). A number of studies highlight that women's individual experiences of reaching the decision to remain child-free were not as clear-cut as making a choice between discernible options. Instead, they described 'a long, complex, historical process that culminated in living permanently without children' (Morell, 1994).

Sterilization is a decision which destroys any illusion that a woman may eventually come round to the idea of motherhood. A childfree choice effectively creates barriers between women, and some women who are unable to conceive resent the decision by (seemingly) fertile women to give up what others long for. Childfree women are astonished at such attitudes and resent such unwarranted interest and unwelcome interference in what they had believed to be a personal and private decision and, like Jude, commented that they felt themselves to be the target for veiled or openly insulting remarks regarding their 'selfish' nature and other negative personal qualities.

> Very few people know that I have been sterilized. I think it is my business. Occasionally I get asked if I have children and I say, 'no, thank God', and people don't usually pry further. (Christine)

The post-war trend to smaller family size, including the choice to have only one child, has continued. More women appear to be postponing having children until their late thirties and even forties, and research from the Family Policy Studies Centre shows that one in five may go on to remain childfree (Condy, 1995; McAllister, 1998). According to the Family Planning Association (1996), of all the available contraceptive methods in the UK, the oral contraceptive pill has shown a steady rate of use for women aged 16 to 49 years (up from 22 per cent in 1989 to 25 per cent in 1993), with a sharp rise in use by women aged 35 to 39 (from 8 per cent in 1986 to 20 per cent in 1995). Between 1989 and 1995 the proportion of women overall using at least one of the thirteen contemporary contraceptive methods rose from 69 per cent to 73 per cent.

The majority of women who have children, as well as all childfree women who are not sterilized and are intent on avoiding pregnancy, continue to use some form of contraception to regulate their fertility, and they make their choice from the range of currently available methods. The women who delay making a decision to the point in their lives when conception would be difficult or impossible without medical intervention are described as 'postponers' (Morell, 1994) as, until a woman conceives there is no way of checking or knowing for certain whether she is fertile. Women with children who use contraception to guard against any further pregnancies or to space the births of their babies, and women determined to avoid pregnancy at any cost, must treat their bodies in similar ways. As it is necessary for heterosexually active childfree women to take some precautionary measures to prevent conception, many of the diaries and interviews described the necessity of continuing with contraceptive measures as an irritating and increasingly meaningless routine.

A significant misapprehension about childfree women's motives in deciding to be sterilized emerged during discussions with GPs and consultants, and was often posed in the form of a puzzled question: could the women not be bothered to take what are, after all, recognized as efficient and effective contraceptive measures? Yet a very important precipitating factor for people seeking sterilization, despite having tried many methods, was contraceptive problems, particularly with the Pill (Allen, 1985). Other responses from the questionnaire and the interviews show that – without exception – all of the women had used at least one type of contraceptive and, in a number of cases, had tried a wide variety. Both Pauline's and Helen's comments typify the dissatisfaction that childfree women expressed with the methods which are currently available:

> Before sterilization I had tried the Pill (which made me depressed and I put on a stone in weight). The cap (I persevered but found the creams gave me cystitis). The rhythm method (I had an unplanned pregnancy and later miscarried), and lastly the coil (which got lost within the first three weeks and I had to attend hospital for a scan to locate it and have it removed). I did ask to try the Pill again but was refused on the grounds of my age and that I smoked half a dozen cigarettes a day. (Pauline)

> Prior to sterilization I was on the Pill, then the coil, then I got that out, but before I'd decided what to do next I had unprotected intercourse, so I got another coil fitted, then I went back on the Pill. I got fitted for a cap, but it was uncomfortable enough just wearing it never mind having sex with it! I think I may have asked for sterilization again at that point. I was sterilized because I never wanted children in my life and didn't see the point in using

contraceptives for the rest of my fertile life, particularly as nothing is one hundred per cent. (Helen)

Because of modern and developing contraceptive methods and techniques and with a growing awareness of the demands on the earth's resources of an expanding global population, women in the developed countries of the West find themselves confronted by the need to make a decision about motherhood. Most women do have children and some women decide to remain childfree, but ways of reaching such decisions are many and varied and say as much about the social meaning of motherhood to women as does their emotional response to becoming a mother. There did not appear to be one main reason for opting for sterilization, and twelve diarists gave a compilation of reasons (see Appendix) which showed their mistrust and dissatisfaction with currently available contraceptive methods, and also voiced fears about the effects of chemicals on their body.

The Pill as a chemical, and concerns about its long-term use, was specifically mentioned by six diarists and others also mentioned their fear of using anything which was less effective and offered lower protection. Gemma took the Pill before having the operation as she preferred to have 'a semblance of menstrual normality', but she continued to fear that it would fail and she suffered with uncomfortable physical symptoms and mood swings. Sally felt that she had been lucky that a woman doctor at the family planning clinic realized that she did not want children, suggesting that she should come off the Pill and consider sterilization. Although Heather had used the Pill for ten years, until she was 28, the prospect of having to endure a refitting of the IUD 'Copper 7' every two years was enough to reduce her to 'a gibbering idiot'. As a nurse, Sandy had a particular awareness of the problems related to long-term Pill use as well as the benefits.

I never liked taking the Pill. I took it from about age 19 for a few years then stopped, did nothing and had a couple of short-term relationships with unprotected sex. I've never had an abortion or used the morning-after pill but I have had a couple of pregnancy scares when I had unprotected sex. I didn't like the thought of chemicals, pills and potions and I've even considered Norplant (implants) but it's chemicals again and I'm a bit nervous about getting them out once they're in. Condoms are just a nightmare. I wanted something I didn't have to think about ever again. I wanted to be sterilized because I didn't want to keep taking chemicals to control my fertility. My body, my decision! (Sandy)

Some women diarists experienced pregnancy scares during change-overs to other types of pill – usually the mini pill – or found that other medication affected the Pill's efficacy. Even the younger women, brought up with the Pill seeming the obvious choice, had to balance their sexual needs with the risks of conception if they decided to interrupt the monthly routine. Ginny, whose chest infections demanded that she take anti-biotics, knew that contraceptive protection was reduced during the course of treatment and for up to fourteen days afterwards. She lived in fear of getting pregnant, refusing sex with her partner because of the risk of conception and when she developed sickness caused by migraine headaches. Clare also reported years of suffering with severe PMT and thought that part of her discomfort may have been that she did not trust the Pill.

Many other diarists made passing reference to being uneasy with the methods they had relied on for years but not all were unhappy with the Pill: some diaries made no reference at all to side effects or uncertainties. Liz said that the Pill suited her and that she had used it from the age of 18 after having an abortion but that she did not want to stay on it forever. Two months before she was married, Jean considered what she would need and how she would manage contraception and visited her local family planning clinic for the Pill and found that the doctor readily supplied her prescription. A family tragedy in her girlhood was referred to as being part of her reasoning for not wanting children:

I was constantly aware that 'having babies can be dangerous' because of the stillbirth of my sister when I was ten. It was kept quiet and and never talked about after the ambulance in the middle of the night – perhaps the seeds about danger were planted then. (Jean)

After taking the Pill more or less continuously since the age of 19, there were some months when Judith was not in a relationship and there were times when she did not take the Pill nor use other precautions. After Sally's sterilization operation she was pleased that her sex life improved dramatically and felt that her fear of pregnancy may have been more deep-rooted than she had realized. Although women are encouraged to rely on contraception in some form, as being their best hope of avoiding an unwanted pregnancy, a senior consultant had no hesitation in saying that, 'apart from sterilization the only other thing that women could do to be one hundred per cent sure is to practise abstinence' (Consultant B).

Studies show that some childfree women, described as being childless, or not-mothers (Morell, 1994; Bartlett, 1994), identified that being childfree emerged as one of many of the important choices which they made in contemplating their future, and became a part of other decisions in a lifestyle which developed as a result of remaining childfree. They appeared not to have made an initial decision early in life about not having children but lived in ways which made having children unthinkable to them, so that 'childlessness is not understood by these women as a choice but rather as a consequence of choosing to live their present lives' (Morell, 1994).

In this study of childfree sterilized women, however, many of the women who opted for sterilization were very clear that they 'always knew' that they did not want children and planned their lives from a starting point of being and intending to remain childfree. Several women diarists insisted that they did not go through any process in deciding not to have children, and Sally was quite definite that there was no one point at which she made a choice: 'I just never saw myself as having children therefore I didn't decide not to have them'. Jill said that the decision to be childfree and the later decision to be sterilized were years apart: 'being sterilized wasn't anything to do with knowing I was not going to have children – I'd always known that I wasn't – it was just the best way of bringing that about'.[2]

Over a quarter of a decade later, Sally and Jill are echoing the words of a woman sterilized in her mid-twenties and who wrote about her decision and experience:

> When I first decided to get sterilised, at twenty-five, it seemed the natural outcome of a lifetime of not wanting children. I had no thoughts of the immorality of overpopulation, or of a woman's duty to define herself outside the traditional area of the home. I simply had never much enjoyed being around children, and saw no reason to spend a major part of my life with them. (Karen Lindsey in Dowrick and Grundberg, 1980, 243)

When writing about their career and life plans, most diarists emphasized that whilst they always knew that they did not want children this
was not necessarily because of a burning ambition to do something else
which motherhood would have prevented. Linda L. appears to fit the
stereotype of a successful and ambitious career woman, but her view of
herself is much more down-to-earth:

> I didn't have a grand plan for my life. I'm a personal assistant,
> quite small fry really, but I enjoy my job and get a lot out of it. I
> know quite a few people without children and I'll be interested to
> see the ratio in ten or fifteen years time. I definitely think that
> there's some sort of change as more people my age are making the
> choice never to have children. Women who get higher up the
> career ladder feel they're in stronger, more secure positions in their
> jobs. The job market is much wider now and women are aware
> that they don't need a man to prop them up. Once you had to have
> a man who had real earning power – now women have that power.
> (Linda L.)

Sally's interview revealed that her early life allowed her the opportunity to travel: 'well, I didn't have a particular ambition – I bummed about
Australia for a while – I just wanted to see life and do things'. She was able
to drift and took pleasure in being flexible and having the freedom to be
responsive to different experiences. Anne T. was aware of wanting
something different for her future life and foresaw restraints on any
future ambitions she might have – even those which had not yet become
clear – because of what seemed to be very negative aspects of motherhood:

> I didn't have a particular life ambition – if there was one, children
> weren't part of it! The very strong message when I was a girl was
> that if you got pregnant it was the end of your life. When I got
> married I realized it was possible to work and have children, but I
> just never wanted to – although I never told my mother! (Anne
> T.)

A few diarists recalled that they had taken some time to consider their
reasons for making the choice. These realizations were slower to emerge
and, rather than saying that they had 'always known', the women
acknowledged that their decision emerged over a period of time. Sandy

had dreams of having loads of kids when she was a child but 'as soon as I hit maturity at about 18, I was aware that I did not want kids. I remember dreaming that I was pregnant when I was in my early twenties and I was terrified. That was when the feeling I didn't want kids really gelled.' Like most young married couples, Linda R. and her husband planned their early life together on the basis of their income. There was no definite plan not to have children but they did not allow the issue just to drift on, 'periodically we reviewed the situation and decided we were happy as we were'. The urge to have a child had been quite strong for Heather and she wrote that she could not pinpoint exactly when she made the decision not to have children as the change was so gradual; 'as a youngster I was crazy about babies and little kids. I was always borrowing babies to wheel out in big shiny prams and then babysitting for all the neighbours. As I got older the urge just sort of faded.'

Personal and social contexts for remaining childfree

A number of the social, cultural and economic changes which have taken place in post-war Britain have been significant for women determined to make personal decisions relating to their future lives. Women themselves vigorously contribute to change through their active agency and, far from being passive, many actively intervene in diverse ways and at complex social levels, perhaps for themselves and their communities, or to bring about more fundamental social, political and economic changes (Charles, 1993). Compared with only a few decades ago, women now occupy different places and perform a wide variety of roles in contemporary British society, although feminists and social commentators are generally agreed that there is still a long way to go.[3]

Although women may now be having fewer children, and having them later in life than historically has been the case, reproductive choices are highly circumscribed and it appears to be a compulsory state which women are expected to enter (Hanmer, 1993) and most women do so via marriage or permanent domestic arrangements and relationships in which they and their partners and children create a family. Because the experience for most people is of living in a family of some type, feminist research has focused on the pressures which exist within what feminists of many persuasions see as 'the site of gender struggle' (Humm, 1989).

Black feminists, however, have criticized white feminist assertions for assuming that the family has universal characteristics and that the nature of the family is necessarily oppressive. In the developing world there are aspects of family which, both historically and in contemporary life, have provided safety and opportunities for self-determination in an otherwise exploitative world. This criticism and others have posed a steady and irresistible challenge to the traditional 'cereal-packet' image of the normal family (Jackson, in Richardson and Robinson, 1993), with its white middle-class heterosexual couple, breadwinner husband, dependent homemaker wife, and their two children: one boy, one girl.

The profile of contemporary family units in Britain includes same-sex households; single householders; unmarried couples; multiple divorces leading to complex childcare arrangements; culturally diverse households, and those which reverse what is considered to be traditional, with the woman as the main earner of the family income and the man as house-husband and child carer. The Cairo Conference in 1994 rejected the insistence of the Vatican and other fundamentalists that there was any such thing as a family structure which could be universally recognized as 'normal' (Petchesky, 1995), emphasizing many times and in many ways that there is a rich global diversity of family forms.[4] These modern realities are no longer predicated only on a narrow view of the nuclear family, a situation which has been described as an 'ideology of household organisation, kinship relation and sexuality' (Chandler, 1991), although politicians and governments continue to create legislation and make references to the family as though it has remained unchanged from an imagined past stability.

However, despite an increasing mismatch between idealized norms and reality, the family continues to provide a major definition of women so that 'women are either married or they are not' (Chandler, 1991), and at the point at which a woman makes the transition from being single to being married she becomes a target for the type of advice and comment – including from family members, other women and cultural and media representations – about what is expected of her in taking on such a role. In many social and cultural contexts, marriage is seen to confer status, but that does not mean that women are able to operate more freely as agents in control of their own fertility and reproductive choices. Instead, the continuing childless state of a young married woman will draw open and critical comment from others, especially if no babies are produced after several years, and a married couple who remain childless are viewed and spoken of with disapproval:

> Selfish, immature, irresponsible, unnatural, inadequate: these are just some of the words which may be used to describe women who choose a childless or, more positively, child-free marriage. (Richardson, 1993, 64)

For some young women the achievement of womanhood is via the status of marriage and aspirations to motherhood (Friedan, 1963; Phoenix, 1991). Part of this transition may also be to behave like 'real' women who express a wish for and want babies, and then go on to have them: for some women there is no question that 'parenting is the embodiment of what an adult is' (Kaplan, 1992). Research into women who are on the margins of marriage shows that the vital importance of being married is a keynote message given to women during early life and, whether or not she marries, it is a major feature in women's lives and the unmarried become stigmatized (Chandler, 1991). Similarly, childbirth and children are important issues for all women, whether or not they go on to become mothers (Trebilcot, 1983) and the term 'maternal thinking' is used to describe a facility which all women possess because of the capacity to reproduce and rear children (Ruddick, 1980). Some feminist writers believe that what cannot be discounted are the ways in which female children become women through gendering during socialization, and contact with all things female and maternal (Mitchell, 1966; Belotti, 1975; Sharpe, 1976; Chodorow, 1978).

Figures from UNFPA show an annual estimate of thirty million births of children whose conception was unwelcome and unwanted. Women who have had children may have planned and wanted them, or they may not. They may have wished for one child but had more, or planned for several but had only one. In order to achieve at least one boy or one girl, women may have more children than they thought they wanted.[5] Some women may be sorry to have had any children at all or have several which were planned but – perhaps secretly – later regretted. Having limited themselves early in life to one boy–one girl, they may choose to have a third child relatively late in life, when their other children are young adults; and not all women can or do conceive. Some women may be too young or too old (in terms of their fertility potential); may identify as lesbian (those choosing not to have a child); may be celibate or otherwise not heterosexually active; may have some challenge or disability, and prefer not to have children for these reasons rather than being voluntarily childfree; or although potentially fertile themselves, may be with infertile male partners or partners who in some way are incompatible with them in terms of their being able to conceive.

Greater interest in the problems of infertility for individuals and research into reproductive technologies and innovative contraceptive methods has increased medical and social concerns for the involuntarily childless and highlighted the distress of women who have problems conceiving a longed-for child. The sympathy and commiseration extended to the estimated one in six of the population who experience difficulties in conceiving or carrying a baby to full term shows the concern of a society which, theoretically at least, considers that it is every woman's right to be able to bear a child of her own (Warnock, 1984). Organizations such as ISSUE (previously the National Association for the Childless) offer support for the grief and desolation experienced by those who assumed that a child would be part of their life, tried to become pregnant and (in their own terms) have failed. However, sympathy and concern is not extended in every case to those who are involuntarily childless: indeed, for those who seek infertility 'treatment' there may be judgement by medics, hostile questioning by media and embarrassed silence, or a pitying attitude, by family, friends and colleagues.

Much feminist research acknowledges that many women do not experience their lives as oppressive, and recognize that they are only rarely totally powerless, yet Gayle Letherby's doctoral thesis (Letherby, 1997) identified that 'infertile' or 'involuntarily childless' women feel that they are excluded from certain situations in society. The women that she interviewed spoke of feeling 'isolation' (Emily), 'inferior and different' (Belle) and the telling comment, 'Members of the club to which I don't belong swap stories' (Frannie). In this way, there is a commonality of experience in that involuntarily childless women and electively childfree women may feel that they are perceived as different, or even abnormal (this is explored further in the following chapter).

Women have always sought to have children if they have been unable to conceive and, traditionally, this was often through adoption, but rapid developments and new technologies in infertility treatment and in the more open practice of surrogacy present some opportunities for achieving motherhood if this cannot occur through what is considered to be the natural process of heterosexual sex, conception, pregnancy and child-birth. Government reports and research by healthcare professionals revealed not only the developments in reproductive technologies but also uncovered the moral dilemmas, such as embryo experimentation, which have emerged as a result of concerns (Fromer, 1983; Warnock, 1984). Other research, more critical of such developments, warns of the impact of these new technologies on women's lives, especially the consequences of the masculine desire to control the creation of life (Rowland, 1992) and the important questions which are raised about women's repro-ductive choices (Greer, 1984; Rowland, 1992; Richardson, 1993). Media reports and debates on the subject give sympathetic coverage of involun-tary childlessness, and to hear women without children speaking about and comparing what they describe as the emptiness of their lives to the lives of women with children is also to discern that there are substantial divisions between them. These divisions appear to be perpetuated and reinforced by the centuries-old message that the function that defines a woman is that she produces children: if she cannot, then she is not a real woman (Corea, 1988).[6]

The motherhood continuum: mothers and not-mothers

The influence of motherhood on women's lives and identities makes it appear that women who have no children seem to be not as normal as women who do and, in many cultures, women have little or no status if they forgo having a man's children or if they are unable to produce a child. If it is the case that there is little to separate the meanings and concepts of motherhood and womanhood, and that they are taken to mean the same thing, then there are implications for women who will not – rather than cannot – bear children. Women are under intense pressure to become mothers and also to care for others, and a leading world patriarch has made the global pronouncement that for women to achieve true liberation 'they need only to recognise that their specific, feminine vocation is to become a mother' (Pope Paul V, 1972, in Daly, 1978). By positioning childfree women as deviant and considering them to be of lower worth compared with women who have or want children, the association of womanhood with motherhood is maintained. Any woman without children is then in danger of being defined as defective (Trebilcot, 1983), therefore not as normal as other women.

> [the work] of 'normalizing' motherhood is carried on through the production and distribution of discourses that depreciate childless women. In this way the modern construction of deviance works to create hierarchies among women based on reproductive differ-ence. (Morell, 1994, 15–16)

Despite an almost universal assumption that it is normal for all women to have children, the briefest examination exposes the pressures and defining boundaries of cultural expectations. For example, very young women, women approaching or beyond the menopause (especially if assisted by some form of medical intervention), single women, or women not in an approved heterosexual relationship, all attract comment and disapproval if they have children. Lesbian and bisexual women are not expected either to want or to have children and may even incur society's wrath and the removal of their children from the family home if they go on to do so. Jude, who is committed to women's rights issues, had noticed that the outrage and shock which accompanied her own decision was not also shown towards those of her lesbian friends who had chosen not to have children. This she felt was 'totally homophobic – it was somehow assumed, without question, that they wouldn't want children anyway, because they are lesbians'.

Women who earn a living from sex work are further trapped within a system which punishes them, the legal system removing children for no other reason than their mother's work. Disapproving comments about the size of their family or generalized remarks about population increases in their country of cultural origin may be made to or about women who are not white, and women with identifiable challenges such as Down's Syndrome may have to undergo abortion or sterilization if they become pregnant[7] and those charged with making decisions for them, usually their parents or social and medical carers, will use their own criteria to consider the life and circumstances and what is in the best interests of the woman and then act upon these conclusions.

It is possible to identify an important contradiction, which appears to be that there is encouragement and an expectation that some women will have children, whilst certain other women may be disapproved of and even prevented from doing so. Women are not equally able to make a choice about having children, for one of the strong social beliefs about motherhood is that only women in stable heterosexual relationships should be encouraged to become mothers (Richardson, 1993). Thus, there are women who are not heterosexual; not married or in a monogamous relationship with a man and who intend to remain single; differently-abled women; women deemed to be sexually promiscuous; women sex workers; or women who otherwise do not conform to her culture's image of what a mother must be. All of these factors tend to single women out for criticism if they go on to have children.

The diary entries and the illuminating and enlightening discussions with childfree women in this study highlighted that there are problems with permanently positioning all women in relation to motherhood. The concept of a 'motherhood continuum' (Rich, 1976) appears to offer a broad sweep to include all women, even though it excludes and has no easy place for the active rejection by some women of motherhood as part of their womanhood and those who may not accept Rich's assertion of reproductive obligations as being as personally relevant. Some writers do not see this conceptual continuum as dangerous to the notion of 'woman' being a complete entity without children. For example, in her defence of the motherhood continuum, Joyce Trebilcot acknowledges the importance of the concept, emphasizes that mothering is central to every woman in patriarchal contexts, regardless of whether or not we are mothers or have the care of children, and posits that it must continue to be a necessary focus for work in feminist theory (Trebilcot 1983).

There is danger in this approach, however. Contemporary feminism continues to smooth over the clear and very obvious differences between women who are and women who are not mothers, but there are calls for a feminist analysis of women's experiences of non-motherhood, one which should be concerned with new ways of defining this experience (Letherby, 1994). Based on the personal experience of being a woman who is involuntarily childless, Gayle Letherby suggests that, as feminist inquiry gets to grips with this fundamental difference between women, a greater understanding of the lives of all women who do not mother children will lead to a wider understanding of female experience, including definitions of women's self-identities. Yet, rather than account being taken of the embracing nature of Adrienne Rich's thinking about a motherhood continuum, which allows for women's location at any point, what appears to happen is that women are assigned to one of only two categories: mother, or not-mother. When separations of this nature occur, one inference is that within the discourse there has been a polarization in feminist thinking, in which women fall into one of these two camps. Instead of using the notion of a motherhood continuum, therefore, what may happen is that women experience a 'motherhood divide' which may have the effect of separating and dividing women as mothers or not-mothers, sometimes even against each other.

A number of examples from the diaries highlighted what may be considered to be experiences of the hierarchies based on and operating around the reproductive differences between women (Morell, 1994). It appears that, because of their great desire to conceive, some women cannot comprehend the motivation or seeming ease with which fertile women make choices about not having babies, with opportunities for access to abortion for unwanted pregnancies setting up additional tensions. However, women who had had children were also unsettled by women who have none and responded in ways which seems to illustrate that they consider childfree women as not normal. The diarists described being personally involved in situations in which they encountered fury and verbal aggression directed towards them by other women who were mothers as well as those without children.

Sally wrote and spoke strongly about her affection for nieces and nephews and the children of friends and was always forthright in any discussions with family or friends about her decision to remain without children, yet she also encountered attitudes which were distinctly hostile, saying that 'women generally act quite aggressively particularly if they have children themselves'. Such accounts were a feature of a number of interviews and their writing also showed hurt and anger – and often incomprehension – that other women could demonstrate such resentment and antagonism towards them. As some of the hostility directed towards women who are voluntarily childfree comes from women who are eager to have a child, Helen, like Jude and a number of the other diarists, spoke of feeling the need to defend her decision:

> Since the operation I have tripped over people who are unable to have children (including my oldest friend for over 20 years) and it seems incomprehensible to them that I should so 'capriciously' give up what they so desperately want. I continually have to justify my choice. (Helen)

Judith was painfully aware of the way that she may appear to other women who wanted to have children and her successful application for sterilization resulted in a hospital experience in which she felt isolated by her childfree status and choice.

> I tried to avoid getting into conversations in the hospital as there were also women in there who were desperate to have children, or were having infertility treatment or trying to get sterilization reversed. I think one woman was recovering from a miscarriage. I kept my head in a book or was knitting most of the time, but had to mingle at lunchtime. I had made a choice that most felt incomprehensible and a couple of women were really not able to talk to me once they knew why I was there. Most seemed to respect my decision even if they thought I was crazy! (Judith)

For Ginny, the most difficult part of the decision to remain childfree was in dealing with the reaction from the traditional element within her Church. She described much sorrow and tension in this important area of her life, particularly as she felt that she is perceived by some to be a wrongdoer.

> The biggest problem was with my religion. They seem to think people come to this earth to get married and have children . . . I have even been told by several women in my Church that I am evil and this is Satan's talk about my decision to be childfree. (Ginny)

The life experiences which separate women who have children and childfree women range from the environments of work and social events to the physical experiences of the birth and the adjustments which are a necessary part of becoming a mother. Once pregnant, a woman is required to make choices – albeit limited – such as, for example, how long she will continue in employment and paid work, or how much time she will take for antenatal appointments and whether she feels that it will be useful to attend birth preparation sessions. Additionally, her social life will be restricted as she moves into the later stages of pregnancy, as she will have other responsibilities and calls on her time and may wish to rest more. This latter may be a component of what have been described as 'friendship wedges' and are characterized by the deviating interests and lack of availability of the soon-to-be mother (Morell, 1994). Pregnant women have unique experiences to which childfree women will have no access unless they work in the medical field (and even then only as observers). The language of those experiences is inclusive (between mothers and to-be mothers) as well as exclusive (of childfree women), with references to physical symptoms (bodily changes), fears and assurances (pain, which other mothers assure will be soon forgotten), wise-woman lore and superstitions (carried high, it is a boy, carried low, it is a girl, or some such variant) and practical advice on feeding, handling, clothing and rearing, which forms part of the initiation into motherhood and is conducted by women, for women.

Once born, children monopolize the lives of couples and, whether or not they are actually present – for example, at a dinner party or other social event – topics about and around children often dominate adult conversations because of the impact on the lifestyles, time and travel plans, household budgets and economic planning, of their parents. Childfree couples become excluded from the social rituals of planning for school runs, parents evenings and birthday parties, and often experience annoyance or boredom as previously well-established friendships change and are affected by the demands of family life. Because of the intimate nature of female friendship, women sometimes feel left out, or left behind, once a friend also becomes a mother (Morell, 1994) and further divisions are created by mothers who believe the subject of their children to be the most fascinating in the universe: the daily life of mothers with the exchange of details about their children is one which is most boring to childfree women (Shapiro, in Morell, 1994).

No matter how tedious those who are childfree may find such contact, however, some involvement with the rituals of motherhood is necessary for most parts of social life, mainly because most women are mothers.

> When I attended a religious group other women often spoke about babies and milk and feeding and burping – it was all blood, sweat, and milk! – but at least they taught me to speak that language so I could 'pass' as a real woman. I'm afraid that if a childfree woman doesn't talk the language, then she doesn't pass among other women as real. If I hadn't learned to speak that language then I would have been a reject. (Vicky)

Motherhood comes about in many ways, not all of which are positive or welcomed. Women become pregnant through failed contraception, or by not using protection and taking chances or any combination of situations which they may describe as 'just bad luck'. Additionally, the violences against women cannot be ignored, and rape, incest and coerced sex may also lead to unwanted pregnancy. The unequal and uneven provision of freely available and effective contraception and lack of uncomplicated access to safe abortion adds to the complex profile of a 'motherhood continuum' which attempts to encompass the many ways that women deal with their reproductive lives. Such diversity in women's experiences and the divisions that may be created between mothers and not-mothers are only part of the wider picture of their lives.

There were obvious inconsistencies in people's perception of them-selves as parents and their ready opinions of Sandy's decision not to have children. These were not lost on her and she found some of the attitudes a source of private amusement, especially when she also detected envy.

> Some people said that children were the most important thing in their lives – but they didn't talk that way to the kids themselves, always telling them off, or complaining how they were draining the life out of them. A couple of people admitted that they wished they hadn't had kids, and envied me! (Sandy)

Most women deal individually and appropriately with any strains which arise in social encounters and friendships so that situations remain on an even keel and, although sometimes anger and resentment erupt, communications generally remain open and are at least tolerable. How-ever, even where these do not present insurmountable barriers to everyday relationships, there are tangible and noticeable tensions between women who can have children, those who cannot and the minority who do not and will not, which cannot be addressed or explained by reference to Adrienne Rich's all-embracing motherhood continuum. All heterosexually active women who have or want children must be conscientious and vigilant with contraception if they are to space the births of their babies, but for childfree women contraception is not intended to delay, or postpone or temporarily avoid pregnancy. Rather, it is a deliberate and concerted attempt permanently to prevent their body's inexorable momentum towards conception. The most used phrase by the diarists was 'I've always known that I didn't want children' and this strength of feeling ran as a theme throughout the written diary entries and was reiterated and returned to again and again during the interviews.

Postponing, shelving or permanently preventing

In Britain, the average age at which a woman has her first child has risen to 27-plus, although what seems to have been a postponement of mother-hood is also now showing with women in the 35-plus age range. Many women who say that they experience an 'overwhelming urge' to have a baby find this emotional force so unexpected that they feel that it comes out of nowhere. For some women it cannot be ignored and will not be shelved indefinitely; 'the question of whether to have children hits people differently at different points in their lives' (Michelene Wandor, in Dowrick and Grundberg, 1980), which also highlights that, for most women, the 'motherhood question' is not answered by a once-and-for-all decision.

> As I am 59 now the Pill wasn't around in my early life and we had to rely on condoms. There were a few scares, and I felt awful as I didn't want a child then. I didn't look at my friend's babies and think 'Oh, I want one . . .' but I did get to various stages when it was just this deeply emotional feeling – an urge towards having a child. (Jane)

One of the anthologies of women writing about their own feelings about motherhood and children contained several accounts of how perceptions of becoming mother are original and diverse between women: those who say simply, 'I want a child', going on to explore and verbalize that statement in ways which highlight their individual motiva-tion behind the 'I want . . .':

> I lusted after a baby exactly as I had lusted after beautiful lovable adults. I wanted a child, a family of my own, someone to need and want me: and also, I wanted to do that thing, called pregnancy and childbirth, with my body – my own beautiful and brilliant wom-an's body. I saw children as an essential part of my deliberate and clear plan for my own life. (Maitland, in Dowrick and Grundberg, 1980, 77–91)

Sara Maitland tells a 'love story', with her daughter as the central character, despite strongly disapproving of romantic love and acknowl-edging the complex, other emotions which are also stirred. She continued,

I know that the feelings that I have for her respond more nearly to the women's magazines / mediaeval poet's / religious mystics' descriptions of love than anything else I have ever felt. I find my daughter movingly, passionately beautiful: when I see her running naked, or coiled sleeping . . . [yet] Emotionally, psychologically, politically, socially, my daughter has forced unwelcome changes on me . . . and I chose that oppression, and do not regret it; indeed, I embrace it with love and joy. (Ibid.)

Unlike the majority of other women, childfree women have no breaks for childbearing and rearing and extend the period of contraceptive use to the end of their fertile lives. A minority of this minority of voluntarily childfree women go on to opt for sterilization as their answer to ceasing to use chemical and barrier contraceptives and see sterilization as the conclusive way of ensuring that choice cannot be compromised by contraception failure.

As well as identifying the various and unpleasant physical side effects or the problems and difficulties in using some of the methods – particularly the cap, or IUDs – the diarists were anxious about the possibility of pregnancy and the distress of having to undergo termination if they were to remain childfree. Sandy's terse 'My body, my decision . . .' also referred to the way in which most of the women determined not to relinquish their complete control over the personal decision never to have children. Whether in a relationship at the time of making the decision and undergoing the operation, or moving out of, or between relationships, or being in one which was temporary and transitory, and regardless of the opinions or attempted influences of a husband or partner, most of the diarists emphasized and justified the personal nature of the choice. If the male partner had been in agreement and involved this was seen as positive and supportive – but irrelevant. Few of the women had entered into joint decision-making with husband or partner about family planning, nor were they influenced by their partner's wishes and desires for children; if he had been in agreement and involved this was helpful, but ultimately had no bearing on the woman making the final decision.[8] Helen discussed her decision with her husband and friends:

I was sterilized rather than him because I felt more strongly that I would never want children no matter what, whereas he thought that if anything happened to us and he were to partner someone who wanted children then he might father a child in the future. (Helen)

Vicky was relieved when she found that her partner was also dead set against having children even though she quite firmly stated that she could not have been persuaded to have children had he felt otherwise. Jude's decision was made without any reference to her pro-feminist partner, although she acknowledged his support for her choice, and Linda L. wrote:

> I would sum up my personal situation as follows. I never have and do not want children and I have been fortunate to meet a man who both understands why, and also doesn't want children. He has expanded my philosophy on why not! (Linda L.)

For some of the childfree women, being sterilized itself was essential in their personal preferences and conditions, and for entering future relationships and identifying personal boundaries.

> I made the decision to be sterilized because (a) although the Pill suited me I did not want to stay on it forever and (b) although I was not in a relationship it occurred to me that, should I meet someone and he wanted children, there would be a conflict. Sterilization would end the issue and the man concerned would have to make a decision as to whether children were of paramount importance to him and therefore find someone else. (Liz)

Choice and decision-making about contraception is usually (but not always) an integral part of heterosexual relationships and from the 1970s within established marriage or long-term partnerships there has been a growing trend for male sterilization to be considered as the permanent method of contraception for couples, once they believe that their family is complete (Wylie, 1972; Wood, 1974; Fromer, 1983; Allen, 1985). Women who choose and actively seek sterilization, however, may be childfree or already mothers, either in a relationship or living singly. There is little to indicate that many men opt for sterilization unless they have already had children, and the decision about male vasectomy is made when men are part of a couple (Allen, 1985).

For women who are not in a long-term relationship with a man, it is important to make a personal decision about contraception as Judith did for, even though she was living with someone at the time, they both knew that there was no permanent commitment to each other. Although it had not been discussed before marriage, Pauline knew that her husband definitely did want children but she would forestall him by saying there was 'plenty of time'. Christine's problems with contraception and the refusals of her applications for sterilization resulted in several pregnancies and, each time this happened, it crossed her mind that she could be a mother; 'I did consider the pros and cons – but the cons always won'.

As most societies make pervasive efforts to socialize girls into wanting babies when they become women, there is little difficulty in understanding why women should choose motherhood (Richardson, 1993). Few studies (for example, those dealing with the difficulties many women encounter when seeking abortion) provide information on, for example whether and how many of the women who become mothers are reluctant from the outset, or on those who may have preferred to remain childfree or others who continue with a pregnancy despite its unplanned nature. Some women choose abortion, or arrange for other members of the family to rear a child (a traditional form of surrogacy) or give up their baby for adoption and, although infanticide is not perceived as being one of the options used by women in the West, there are sufficient media reports of baby abandonment and babies found dead through neglect after birth or asphyxiation[9] to warrant the belief that such a possibility occurs to a number of desperate women in the UK.

Notes

1. Feminist writers have acknowledged that, as well as the fulfilling, liberatory and enriching elements of becoming a mother, some women find the reality of motherhood to be an oppressive experience for which they had been neither advised nor prepared (Oakley, 1979a; Rowbotham, 1981). None the less, it continues to be the case that for most women the birth of their children and the experience of motherhood is looked forward to with great anticipation.
2. A few of the women commented on the inclusion of my question which requested information about when they 'first knew', or asked why they were being called to account for not wanting children when, to their knowledge, women who did want them were probably not asked the same question.
3. Contemporary surveys (MORI, Social Trends, General Household, for example) show that, despite an almost 50 per cent increase in the number of women managers, they account for only 3 per cent of the total of management posts and that married women or those in live-in partnerships continue to do the greater part of household and domestic duties, often combining this with paid work of some kind.
4. The Cairo Conference: International Conference on Population and Development,

1994: Programme of Action. Reporting on this conference is contained within *UN Chronicle* (September 1994) and (December 1994).

5. A colleague nursery nurse at the school in which I was headteacher told me that she was glad that her mother-in-law was so determined to have a girl that she went on to have eight children. My colleague's husband 'was boy number seven, and number eight was A . . . , the only girl – then she stopped'.

6. During the autumn of 1997 I attended a television programme interview with a 27-year-old woman who had been sterilized at the age of 25. After some rather shallow questioning which was easily dealt with by the young woman, the body-blow question came (I suspect that the chance to ask it was the sole purpose of interviewing her) and she was asked, 'isn't it likely, in fact, that you are just dysfunctional'.

7. As in the case of a 17-year-old woman with 'severe learning difficulties' who underwent enforced sterilization in 1987. The House of Lords agreed that a court decision could be authorized in such a case, where it was considered against a woman's interests to become pregnant.

8. There does seem to be a certain irony implicit within these statements. In the various contexts spoken of by the women, it was their male partners who seemed to be faced with making choices about their potential fatherhood rather than the women being forced into contemplating their latent motherhood.

9. I was writing this at the same time as the appearance of reports in the local and national press of babies who had been abandoned; some were found alive, others were dead. A newborn baby was found two days before Christmas 1996 and was later claimed by a 15-year-old Essex girl. 'Molly' was found abandoned in a hedge in sub-zero temperatures in Gateshead; to date, she remains unclaimed. A 21-year-old Midlands woman was being interviewed by the police after the discovery of a dead baby girl, wrapped in a towel and hidden in a wardrobe; the post-mortem showed that the baby had been born alive but had died later 'from asphyxia'. Post-Christmas 1997, on a housing estate on the outskirts of Birmingham, a 'beautiful newborn baby boy' was found dead, wrapped in a man's jacket, on a pavement outside a block of flats: later reports suggested that he had been stillborn. Such reports are accompanied by appeals for the unknown mothers to present themselves for post-natal care. These appeals are usually in the form of attempting to offer understanding and assurances to the women for, although the police must treat these tragic cases as suspicious deaths, they are always reported with sensitivity and sympathy. I reflected that, for these women, not only the birth but also the whole period of the pregnancy must have been a period of shame, concealment and fear.

Getting off the reproductive bicycle – Chris Eilbeck

'Let me explain', said the female GP. 'The failure rate on the Pill is around 1 in a hundred; it's about 2 in a hundred on the coil and the same for condoms. We recommend the coil as the best alternative to the Pill, if you don't want to take hormones any more, although it has difficulties for women who haven't had children, and the failure rate can be improved by taking hormone tablets with it. Sterilization? About one in 3,500 – but it's difficult to obtain unless you've had children and you're over 40.'

Except for men, of course, who can get it on demand, regardless of age. Perhaps the system wants to prevent young men sowing their patriarchal rights the way we're told they're designed to do. Perhaps there's a secret plan by the NHS to sabotage evolution. Or perhaps the male surgeons want to preserve fertility for themselves.

'You do realize it's irreversible?' asks the gynaecologist, the understanding, liberal gynaecologist, who approves of my Amnesty badge and talks to me as though I were a human being. And then, in hospital, 'You are sure you want to go ahead with this?' They give me a sheet to read.

> Once your tubes have been blocked the effect is permanent. This is the overwhelming disadvantage of sterilization as it is the only form of contraceptive that you cannot stop. [I thought that was the idea, actually . . .] You should not have the operation done unless you are ABSOLUTELY SURE THAT YOU WILL NEVER WISH TO HAVE A FURTHER CHILD.

They believe I am in ignorance of the meaning of the word 'sterilization', despite all their warnings. They believe I think nothing of the risk of taking a general anaesthetic. They believe I think having holes bored through my body is easier than taking pills. And that, when I meet the new man in my life, I will come crying back to a man begging for him to be God and grant me an immaculate conception by the waving of a scalpel. But I don't confuse men with God. I leave that to men.

After the nurse who takes the details and the nurse who takes the blood pressure and the nice, liberal gynaecologist with his avuncular warnings, comes the houseman (who's actually a woman) – to get my signed consent. Underneath my signature is a line for my spouse to sign. The house(wo)man assures me it is not obligatory. Then why is it there? Do many operations require a spouse's consent? No, not many. Are they all operations on women? The NHS does not deign to reply.

4

Personal Choices, Decisions and Medical Responses

I often think, why do I want to be sterilized? The answer is that I believe current contraceptives to be inadequate and I'm not prepared to go through the psychological and emotional trauma of another termination. The plain truth, however, is that I don't want children. I don't consider this a selfish act but an individual response to a social problem. (Emma)

In 'Family Planning' we cannot refer directly – we give accurate information and can only do anything with the GP's consent but there are ways through all systems. Women who don't have accurate information aren't helped by people who say 'You might change your mind'. Sterilization costs a lot, but so what? What about the costs of three or four pregnancies, or several abortions? (Doctor A.)

All women are childfree for some part of their lives and in the West many consciously choose to begin a programme of contraception which they will continue, with greater or lesser success at preventing conception, until they deem the time has arrived for them to begin planning their family and have the first baby. If the chosen method of contraception has been efficient, and has allowed a measure of control over fertility, this usually means deciding to come off the Pill or to stop using the other methods which have delayed pregnancy. Having done so, they have embarked upon the process which many women refer to as 'trying for a baby'. When (and if) the first child has been born, they may recommence with contraception until (and if) it is time to think about the next child.

When women who have chosen to remain without children find that powerful others refuse to countenance the decision to be sterilized then they say that they feel that their own freedom and determination is attacked and may experience a range of negative and undermining emotions: humiliation, frustration, anger and rage, and helplessness. Some speak of having been infantized, not only by the refusal of their request but also through a denial even of their choice to make such a decision:

> A new GP said, 'Oh well, I wonder how many pets you have?' and I can still see his smirk when he asked that. I was eventually sterilized in 1984 and had made enquiries the year before to the NHS but my GP didn't want to refer me. When I finally saw a consultant he laughed at my request and told me to come back when I was married and had had kids. I couldn't believe that I was being ignored in such a way, this was my LIFE he was dismissing . . . Afterwards, I found that I was shaking with anger and cried quite a lot in the toilets. (Anne D.)[1]

Such an experience has much in common with that of pregnant women who, according to Ann Oakley, are considered and treated as children by many in the medical profession, who hold the belief that it is doctors and not women themselves who are the experts on the subject of motherhood. With reference to much of the 'advice literature' available to women she points out that, 'what is communicated . . . is an image of women's essential childishness. They are portrayed as not properly grown-up people . . . beset with distracting whims and foolish fancies.' (Oakley, in Hutter and Williams, 1981). Many of the diarists echoed Anne D.'s fury and feeling of helplessness at being treated as though they were children and, like Emma, expressed exasperation and indignation when told repeatedly by doctors and consultants that they would inevitably come to regret their childfree choice and their decision to be sterilized.

Feminist writers point out that, although the number of women choosing not to have children is increasing, choice is not very meaningful unless it is related to the circumstances of people's lives (Richardson, 1993). Women would be empowered through having the potential to make their own decisions and to exert the power necessary to take control of their own lives, which are often hampered by the nature and structure of society and its systems. Although there are similarities between making choices and making decisions, in philosophical terms no one given choice nor decision has any fundamental right or wrong attached to it, other than that bestowed by social and cultural tradition and practice, for both may be bound up with intentions (Honderich, 1995). Choosing to act in a certain way or to follow a particular pathway leaves other options not chosen: certain doors may then close, perhaps permanently. Later, as a result of making a particular choice over others, consequences neither considered nor foreseen may unexpectedly emerge which, as happened with the diarist Heather (see Appendix), have a profound effect on the planned or expected outcome.

Social and cultural beliefs and convictions about women's disposition, their choices and decisions, appear so normal that they are seldom questioned and one strongly held belief is that all women want children, and will feel incomplete if they do not have one. So strong is this, that women without children who wish to end any future possibility of motherhood are seen as having made an irrational choice. In the unequal relationship between doctor and patient, when the women's decision and request for sterilization is considered to have no validity and is refused, the reason given is often related to the medic's fundamental belief that no mature woman could reach such a decision and that she will eventually grow out of her infant state, will reach maturity and will then wish to have children.

Other common myths are that women are, or should aspire to be, selfless and self-sacrificing and 'for men' in a sexual, economic and emotional way especially, the myth continues, as women are of lesser intelligence, are less able and not as creative and powerful as men, and in order to fulfil their expected role as good women they 'really ought to be a mother' (Charles, 1993). There is a deeply ingrained association of womanhood with childbearing (Corea, 1985) so that the words woman and mother collapse into a common concept (Morell, 1994). Subscription to a belief in 'maternalism' (a 'femaleness' within which motherly qualities are embedded; Petchesky, in Morell, 1994) and 'maternal thinking' (women having distinctive virtues connected to female mothering; Ruddick, 1982) drives the conviction that women must become mothers if, in traditional Freudian terms, they are also to become complete as women.[2]

Jane acknowledged the difference in herself after her son was born, but this was not necessarily because she felt incomplete or not whole before he arrived, rather that she was still on her personal life journey.

> It's a sort of completeness, but I don't think he defines me as I was a real person before his birth. I've had counselling at various stages in my life and, in retrospect, felt I needed to find myself before I could have thought of having children, or really think about being responsible for another being. (Jane)

The idealization of motherhood and cultural references to a mothering instinct and the confident way in which 'being broody' is talked about and demonstrated by some women is a powerful cultural reference point for pregnancy and motherhood; it appears to be and is accepted as desirable, natural and ultimately normal. Because from infancy women are presented (and some feminists say confronted) with a heterosexual ideal of male penetrative sex as normal sexual activity (Wilkinson and Kitzinger, 1993), the goal and highest achievement of womanhood is assumed to be the conception of children, joyful pregnancy and radiant motherhood. With a range of contraception only relatively recently becoming widely available and within the reach of more women and, given that in the past untold numbers of women may have considered remaining childfree had such a choice been possible, contraceptive choice has expanded to include not only when, but also whether, to become a mother. This choice is not likely to be one which many women will make, but it has become one of the options which may be considered alongside the others. Only recently have women been able to utilize the diversity of choice and become active agents of their own reproductive decisions which were previously unthinkable, unacceptable and limited by expectations of what it is to be a woman

Whilst it is the case that most women have a child or children, a significant challenge to the idea of a 'mothering instinct' comes from an examination of those women who make a conscious and determined decision against motherhood, and in favour of remaining childfree. A number of the diarists were aware of how they were seen as somehow not real women or, at least, to be lacking in some way: 'My mother's opinion prior to the operation was "no woman can ever be fulfilled until she'd had children" – well, no fulfilment for me, then!' (Pauline). By being a childless woman, Emma felt that her life was perceived as a contradiction and that she became 'an abnormal monster', and Vicky's expression of relief that she had been taught to speak the language spoken by other women who were mothers also signalled her awareness that she would have been rejected on the basis of being a woman without children and could not, therefore, 'pass among other women as real'. For most women, what it is to be a woman and the way in which woman and mother are synonymous exposes a childfree woman as only fulfilling a half of that meaning: because of this, reproductive choice itself may be boundaried and constrained, thus affecting vital aspects of decision-making and lifestyle options.

The search for a word which relates to women who have no children highlights that such women do not have a name: the use of the terms childless, or childfree, emphasizes that they are referred to by what is defined as an absence in their lives.[3] There is a major question regarding what it is to be a mother as well as how to become a mother for, regardless of women's desires and motivation, their racial and cultural identities, sexuality and identity, and even the physical potential for achieving it, motherhood itself is a discourse to be negotiated. Even given maximum choice of alternative lifestyle choices for living without children (safe and sure contraception, secure job and career opportunities, a supportive environment within which such choice would be accepted), the majority of women will continue to choose to have babies, overcoming enormous problems to do so.

In contemporary global terms it remains the case that the majority of women have children and that, even if they desire to limit the number or take opportunities to space those they have, they would not choose to remain childfree. That said, however, for many women it may be more a case of bad timing which precipitates entry into motherhood as often as a whole-hearted decision to have a child. Risk-taking, as well as contraceptive failure, often accompanies heterosexual activity and may result in an unplanned pregnancy, so that for many women it is then not so much a case of having made a decision to conceive as the decision being made for them. At that point, and if she has any choice in making such choices, a woman may continue with or terminate a pregnancy, basing her decision on personal considerations relating to lifestyle expectations, economic and career pressures, and domestic and partnership concerns. If she opts for abortion it may be more for a 'not now, not this one' reason rather than a 'not now, not ever' decision.

One of the most important social institutions which profoundly affects all individuals is the field of medical practice and research. The medical profession has been criticized by feminists and agencies providing birth control advice and support for preventing women from fully managing their own fertility so that women say that they feel disempowered from controlling this vital area of their life. Doctors and specialists are increasingly interested and involved in the reproductive technologies for infertility at the same time as refusing or delaying abortion or elective sterilization procedures. This lays doctors open to the charge that they continue to control not only those who will have children but also those who will not. In part through Marie Stopes's eugenics-based legacy, the enthusiasm of population controllers for sterilization programmes in the developing world attracts critical examination when compared with the demonstrated reluctance of doctors in the West to agree to applications for sterilization from childfree women.

Many women conceive despite their precautions and convictions. Contraception may be inadequate or fail, or unprotected or unwanted sex – including rape – may result in an unwelcome pregnancy. At this point the childfree women may decide that the time has come for her to act upon her decision not to have children, opting for termination and sterilization in one fell swoop, but there was clear consensus amongst professionals that sterilization is not appropriate at a time of crisis or considerable change (Allen, 1985). In a written response to a question about reversal rates of sterilization a leading specialist was clear: 'patients who were sterilized at the time of a pregnancy were much more likely to regret the operation . . . ' (Professor Lord Robert Winston, personal letter, 13 Dec. 1996). Several of the women's diaries suggested that this was not so in their case. Gillian was refused sterilization, became pregnant and then had the sterilization and termination together, and has no regrets other than feeling angry that the pregnancy was the result of her application being ignored.

I was sterilized in 1976 (aged 26) three months after we got married. My tubes were tied in case I wanted the procedure reversed due to my age and the fact that I had no children. I had the operation through the BPAS – I got pregnant so had a termination at the same time. I was waiting for an appointment for the NHS and failed contraception led to this. (Gillian)

Most of the childfree women commented that they had felt that their decisions were ignored or trivialized and their well-considered and rational reasons for choosing sterilization were compromised. They regarded this as being exposed to the risk of unwanted pregnancy especially where they were already vulnerable through changes in their contraceptive methods or because their age prompted doctors to advise alternatives to the Pill.

[There was also clear evidence that] women who were perfectly happy on the pill, with no apparent health problems, were being advised by doctors to come off it, sometimes at the age of thirty. Some of these women were very unhappy about this and, considering that some of the consultant gynaecologists felt that it was often better to continue on the pill rather than have a sterilization, there did appear to be a difference of opinion over the advisability of sterilization. (Allen, 1985, 13)

Some found that their applications for sterilization were turned down or delayed for so long that they became pregnant, necessitating immediate and painful decisions. Vicky used the common term 'scare' to describe a monthly experience for many women of wondering whether their contraception had let them down: 'The scare happened just as I was changing to the mini pill. I remember being terribly worried that I might be pregnant, and then relieved that I wasn't.' The same term was used by Anne D., who said that she, 'was on the Pill on and off until I was sterilized. I did have a couple of scares and these were very stressful times when I felt even more helpless and out of control.'

Christine, who also had no regrets at having an abortion and sterilization at the same time, gave a harrowing account of her experiences of refusals, and suggested that her needs as a patient were ignored to an extent which bordered on cruelty.

I have been pregnant four times. The third time I went to BPAS I did mention the possibility of being sterilized but I was told no, as it wouldn't even be considered in someone so young. When I went the fourth time and said I wanted to be sterilized the doctor said it was a bit drastic. I said, 'So is having four abortions!', then it was agreed that I could have the sterilization as well as the abortion. That was eleven years ago and I have never regretted either the decision or the operation. (Christine)

Several other women felt that they had been put in such a situation and breathed a sigh of relief when they realized that the scare was a late period. These accidents and scares were referred to several times as the 'final straw' by women reporting years of using unsatisfactory contraception.[4] Some women who experienced an unplanned pregnancy chose abortion: others reapplied for sterilization and became even more determined to succeed.

After using alternative contraception and having a 'scare' I thought – right, that's it! I said to the doctor, 'I'm not pregnant this time and I want to make an appointment for next week to talk about sterilization'. (Linda L.)

The British Pregnancy Advisory Service was set up and developed in direct response to an absence of facilities for young, unmarried people which became evident during the initial years of what has come to be known as the 1960s sexual revolution and, even now, appears to be in the vanguard of progressive thinking about sexual behaviour when compared with the more cautious approach shown in some cases by people in the medical profession. Neither in their literature nor in personal discussion is there overt evidence of any moralistic tone when having to confront contentious issues which cause problems in the wider society.

The services provided by BPAS are not age limited, we will see any young person and our clients are probably those under twenty-five. We take everyone seriously and have advice sessions for clients aged from eleven or twelve who are sexually active. They come because they haven't been able to get what they want elsewhere or feel uncomfortable about talking to their GP. Some young women come who don't see themselves ever having a family, and we don't laugh at them or send them away. Now, this is going to get terribly politically incorrect – and it is a personal statement, definitely not a BPAS understanding – but I feel that a lot of male doctors confronted by a young woman who doesn't want children would find such a thing difficult. Well, they'd think, it's a gift – they can reproduce if they choose to and a man can't. It's generally thought that if a woman has got the 'kit' then she should use it. (Senior member of staff, Midlands BPAS branch)

Age is a further crucial factor when a woman applies for sterilization and, once again, women feel that they are not taken seriously until an accident or scare precipitates a traumatic decision. Although there is a general feeling of social disapproval as well as legal restrictions, early sexual activity information and advice about contraception is essential if heterosexually active young women are to avoid pregnancy. For some women, however, it seems that the advice given to them is less than helpful in achieving control over their fertility and they are forced to seek an alternative to the family GP in making their request. Jude wrote that not only had she always known that she did not want children but also 'I knew that I actually wanted to be sterilized and asked my doctor when I was eighteen'. As with Emma's applications, such a young age is never seen by doctors to be appropriate for making long-term decisions of this nature, although sympathy was expressed for the problems and frustrations expressed by women whose applications were unsuccessful:

I feel sorry for women who really feel that they want sterilization. I'm sure that it would be helpful if they could see someone who could say 'Well, at twenty-five you're on the borderline of not being able to make up your mind finally and fully, but come back in three months'. I would never say two years – somebody who has a problem has it NOW, they need to talk NOW about it – and they usually can't get that by talking to their GP, so I'll keep seeing them and I'll document each time they come, so eventually they will get what they want. (Family planning nurse)

Women who are determined to have no children are also intent on avoiding pregnancy at any cost, and so there are serious problems if doctors and consultants are overly cautious in their willingness to take their sterilization requests seriously. If doctors are suspicious of a woman's motives and decide to adopt an approach which verges on the psychological, there will be delay and the danger of an unplanned pregnancy.

> Now, objectively, it is much more likely that someone with no children clearly might want to have it undone and might regret the decision, therefore you have to be much more . . . well, stringent, perhaps, in discussion with them to make sure they really appreciate what they are doing. At each point of referral there are hurdles and 'dropping-off' points and that could be a good or a bad thing so that these may be seen as barriers put in the way to put people off, but they may test their resolve, for example, if they're doing this for some temporary emotional upset . . . I mean, what sort of statement is the person trying to make by doing this? (Consultant A.)

It appears that there are complex medical and ethical decisions to be made when sterilization is being requested by an otherwise healthy woman rather than when it is medically necessary. However, women who say that they have 'always known' that they do not want children feel that the decision which has taken them sometimes years to reach, often in the face of hostility, and usually after a great deal of determination in getting as far as seeing a consultant, should not be dismissed as though it were a temporary aberration. Women who do not want to become mothers also do not want to become pregnant and such a testing of resolve, at the point which women might expect to be the final hurdle, may be seen instead as a final dismissal. Later in this interview the same consultant demonstrated much sympathy and concern for patients, his initial stringency modified and tempered by his personal and professional guidelines for acting on initial requests.

> I have a responsibility to check that they have thought it through, and to go through a process, a little counselling, so they and I know what's happening. I'm not trying to put them off, or be judgemental, but – and back to my original guideline – they shouldn't do something they'll regret. It's never an easy decision, we're usually condemned whichever way we go – I'd say that there is no ultimate 'right' or 'wrong' decision (Consultant A.)

This considered approach was the position which I heard from all of professionals that I interviewed and one in which the final stance appeared to be that women's determination will probably get them through in the end – but that there is likely to be no harm done in reining back and not giving immediate approval.

> Generally speaking, medics tend to be very cautious and to some extent they 'run scared' in case they act too soon – they would be anxious about a woman who they have sterilized coming back and saying 'Why did you take me seriously . . .?'. (Senior member of staff, Midlands BPAS branch)

The refusal of a request and application for sterilization was a shock for many of the diarists and many felt humiliated and dismissed. Several spoke in terms identifying that they felt reduced to a state of infancy, although few made an immediate response during their interview with the consultant. Despite initial setbacks, they commented on the necessity of attempting to recover some dignity and also to rally the determination to continue. Emma wrote an impassioned and furious response after being refused for the second time. The disastrous consequences of the past failure of contraception and a traumatic abortion left her feeling that she faced a bleak future, and would have to struggle with unsatisfactory attempts at contraception until reaching the age of 30: even then she was not confident of making a successful application. Her first letter was an outpouring of anger onto the page and was not the one sent to the consultant, but she did eventually write to him and in doing so regained not only a sense of personal dignity but also strength to carry on. She commented that a sense of outrage and indignation may be a strange way for this to come about, but her recovery is well expressed in the post-refusal letter which she did eventually send to the consultant. She did not receive a reply.

> I felt the consultation to be a waste of everybody's time as it was quite clear that we had different opinions on what was best for my future well-being. I do not expect you to change your mind, just as I won't. I am also quite well aware of the political and ideological aspects of reproduction and sexuality which result in women who do not want children being subjected to such experiences whilst those who choose to have children – a decision affecting many more people with far more widespread consequences – are not asked to justify their beliefs or behaviour. (Emma, from a letter to a consultant, November 1996)

In some of the diaries which gave examples of meetings and consultations with GPs and consultants, there was evidence demonstrating real concern for the reasons that women give when requesting sterilization as well as what seemed to be exceptionally liberal attitudes expressed by some consultant gynaecologists. The doctors and consultants interviewed for this study were sympathetic and concerned about women's welfare, yet also anxious about having to juggle the needs, desires and expressed wishes of the patient with their own professional judgement. There was a concern for establishing 'a balance between prohibition and complacency. We have to test people's aims and understanding but not be dictatorial or censorious. I don't have any belief that women should have children – there are already far too many children about – but she shouldn't do something she regrets' (Consultant A.).

Because of the acknowledged lack of research in this area, consultants and GPs generally were influenced by the regrets of a number of women who had been sterilized and wished for reversal: overwhelmingly, these would be women who have had children. Consultants who work in the area of women's reproduction will occasionally have childfree women referred to them and acknowledge that the journey to get so far has likely been long and hard won.

> Women will already have tried all sorts of contraceptives, will have kept pestering their GPs and will already have had a battle before they get to see me. If they have no children I see them myself to take their contraceptive and medical history and I find that the way they come over to me is that they are determined never, under any circumstances, to have babies. After some of the usual information, the small failure rate and what do you do if you meet 'the light-of-your-life' then I say, fine, I'm the technician and you must be prepared to take responsibility for your actions and realize there's no going back, and I write I've told them that on their notes. So then I go through some of the medical and practical aspects and I then say, OK anything else? and they look at me and say, 'do you mean that you'll do it?' When they hear 'yes' they look so happy and relieved – you can tell just by the look in their eyes if they are really convinced . . . and of course they wouldn't have got as far as me if they weren't! (Consultant B.)

A number of women said that they had had positive and helpful experiences and little trouble finding out what they needed to know nor did they experience problems with unhelpful professionals. Anne T. was referred immediately by her male GP and she found that she was able to get the essential and necessary information very easily: 'the process, on the whole, was smooth and untroubled'. When Geraldine was 27 she applied for sterilization via her GP and was interviewed at an NHS hospital in the north-west of England a few weeks later. She decided to decline the admission date and postponed the operation for six months to be absolutely sure and, for her also, the process was smooth 'and none of the professionals gave me a hard time'. Linda L. was pleased to find that the consultant recommended by her GP 'was a really nice guy, he went through the usual "now, have you considered this and that . . . ?"', and she felt fully informed about the various methods of the procedure.

Other childfree women found that they had to wait until their second or subsequent application before discovering that they were taken seriously. Sandy was 32 when she first applied for sterilization as, although she had been aware of the procedure for a number of years, 'I didn't feel it was worth trying when I was younger'. The consultant knew her but she gained no priority or special treatment because of this; instead 'he struck a bargain saying come back in a year's time. In the end, I waited two years for the NHS operation, one month short of my thirty-fifth birthday.' Similar in age to Sandy, Jean also first asked to be sterilized at 32, but 'the woman GP just refused as she said she didn't think women without children should be sterilized'. Later, when discussing with a male GP her fears about the long-term issue of being on the Pill she found that she was facing 'a two-year waiting list, or going private for £2,000'.

There was no obvious difference in attitude demonstrated between male or female medical practitioners and the diary entries showed that women doctors were just as likely as male doctors and specialists to display dismissive and patronizing attitudes and behaviour towards childfree women wanting sterilization. In a few instances, applicants found that they were dealing directly with consultants who appeared to be expressing personal opinions as part of the argument against sterilizing childfree women.

The consultant was very different from my GP. She came out with the statement that I was only a kid and that I didn't know what I was missing by not having children. When I said that it would interfere with my life and my health was not too good, her reply was that when she was training to be a doctor she had six children! I really argued and she even telephoned a more senior consultant. When she left the room the nurse that was there said to me 'Don't whatever you do give in to them, they will talk you out of it', and that it was my body and I was 31 years old not 21, so I was old enough to make my own decisions. I got it in the end but not only did they try to get me to have the coil instead – I said no way! – but she said I would soon be back to have the operation reversed. (Ginny)

Those who work exclusively within family planning services, however, are more definite about the need to put the woman first even if there are some lingering doubts. Two female family planning specialists, exposed on a daily basis during their work to the anxieties and problems experienced by women in their everyday lives, expressed irritation and exasperation at the way that women were treated on the way to being referred and knew that, even if a childfree woman managed to get as far as a hospital consultant, the response was likely to be that she was much too young and would change her mind. Rather than try to change a woman's mind about what was clearly a firm decision, the family planning nurse used a counselling session to suggest that there were many problems ahead if the woman was intent on waiting for a health service operation.

I feel when in counselling women about what they want that I can't make a decision for her. It's her business, her choice abso-lutely, and I'm here to listen to women. I see a few of these women through the family planning clinic. They definitely do not want to get pregnant and come to a certain age and say 'I know I've not had children but I'm in a stable relationship and I want steriliza-tion – what can I do about it?'. Some will be determined to go for NHS. One said 'I want to prove a point . . . ', but then, of course, there is the risk of pregnancy. It is so frustrating for them. To women who battle against the bureaucracy all the time I'll say, the problem will be solved if you go privately. (Family planning nurse)

She went on to comment that economic considerations play a central role in the decision-making on such applications, as 'we're now working

Trusts and we're talking money. We might say yes but then they go back to the GP who might say "No, I'm not spending my budget on that"': it is important to note that many health authorities will not fund sterilization reversal, under any circumstances. The doctor at the same centre highlighted that there are further and particular obstacles to be overcome if a woman cannot get past a family doctor who may exhibit personal prejudices and be prepared to exert the power of refusal. Doctors hold diverse perspectives and opinions on issues such as antenatal care, contraception and abortion and often that was more to do with the doctor's religion than it was in being a member of the medical profession (Homans, in Homans (ed.), 1985).

> It is awfully difficult to get sterilization, especially for the childless, but for women with children as well. One case I saw recently was of a 25-year-old on her fourth termination after nine pregnancies. I said what I've never said before, 'Why don't you consider sterilization?'. She said that that was just what she wanted – 'I've been asking for years but my female GP, a vicar's wife, said that she "will not permit it", so I can't get anywhere'. Of course, she needs a referral but she agreed with my suggestion to consider a TOP and sterilization at the same time. That was only possible because of the links we can make, but most women don't get further than their GP. She couldn't go private and, well, she just hasn't the 'know-how' to get through. (Doctor A.)

There are clear indications, arising from this study and others, that women's opinions have been disregarded in the past and their preferences dismissed as irrelevant. However, critical changes in attitudes to women's requests, and the ways in which women are perceived and acknowledged as being agents in their own decision-making, are evident in the emerging trend towards more liberal attitudes with a developing tendency for gynaecologists to feel that they should not interfere too much in people's decisions. Isobel Allen's research (Allen, 1985) uncovered markedly different attitudes between consultants, with some saying that they would exercise extreme caution but others giving more weight to the woman's presentation of her decision in their assessment of each particular case, judging each one on its individual merits. One consultant confirmed, 'I do sterilize twenty-one and twenty-two year olds. I don't see why I should say no. I see too many coming back for a TOP at twenty-five saying "Why didn't you sterilize me?".' Another appeared to suggest that his opinions and attitudes had undergone a radical, if reluctant, shift over a period of time: 'I no longer refuse to sterilize patients. I often think they're making a decision with which I disagree but it is their decision' (in Allen, 1985, 244–7).

Responses from consultants for this study, to questions about the changing nature of their gatekeeping role, drew forth similar indications of the ways in which they interpreted and implemented medical thinking and guidelines:

> The rules were much more rigid years ago and we tended not to do anyone under 30 but I've tried to be fairly flexible and change the attitude so as not to put people under too much pressure. I've mellowed with age and also everyone's attitude in the general area of fertility has changed over the years. It's not my job to tell people how to run their lives if they have made a considered decision. It's how people feel inside that's important – some think it's vital to recreate, others just don't want babies whether they have a career or not. (Consultant B.)

The GP that Jill visited 'was so hostile that he reeled back saying that no reputable practitioner would perform such an operation in such circumstances, and as I left he was muttering that "he supposed" it was my body and I could do what I liked – very disapproving!'. In this, her GP appeared to be exhibiting what was identified by the childfree women as a gatekeeper role, allowing subjective opinion and disapproval to show through during the interview and eventually overriding her considered request. This role of gatekeeper is an established and intrinsic part of any doctor's responsibility but may be inappropriate in some situations.

> There is the additional problem that if doctors appropriate the role of decision-makers, and decide that men or women should not be sterilized before a certain age, or before they have had a certain number of children, then sterilization will be inaccessible to the vast number of people who have and want a small family at an early stage of their marriage. They may become eligible in the doctor's terms later on, but it may need a birth or an abortion to act as a catalyst for such a decision and process. (Cartwright, 1976, 169)

An American study which exhorted men and women to opt for voluntary sterilization suggested that sterilization provided the most modern, safe and effective method for birth control (Wylie, 1972). Yet guidelines from the American College of Obstetricians and Gynaecologists on limiting sterilizations included advice to doctors on the way in which they should apply the '120' rule. That is, for a woman even to be considered for sterilization (but not necessarily accepted) a doctor must calculate twice the woman's age, multiply that by the number of her children, and the resulting total must then reach the magic figure of one hundred and twenty. Using this baseline, a woman of 30 with two children could apply and may qualify but no childfree woman could ever be considered during her fertile years.[5] By publishing information on which clinics would carry out sterilizations, and on the basis that there was no legal basis for refusal, Wylie encouraged campaigns and lawsuits against those local laws and hospital administrations routinely denying access to voluntary sterilization. It was, however, generally understood that sterilization in the USA was considered to be appropriate only for married couples, who must both give signed consent, but that married or divorced women or any single women with no children would find most doctors unwilling to recommend anything but contraception (Lanson, 1975).

> my great fantasy developed. [I daydreamed] about being in a terrible car crash and waking up in the hospital [to hear] 'Miss Lindsey, you'll live, but . . . you'll never have children'. And I would shout 'Hooray!' into his startled face . . . I went to my doctor, never doubting that it would be a simple process of announcing my intention and scheduling my operation. My doctor was understanding and sympathetic, but he assured me that no hospital in the country would sterilise an unmarried, childless woman. (Karen Lindsey in Dowrick and Grundberg, 1980, 247)

The International Planned Parenthood Federation reiterated that sterilization is a positive decision, an essential option in the control of human fertility:

> Sterilization as a method of limiting family size is a matter for individual choice which should be made in the full knowledge of alternative methods of contraception and the risks and benefits to health and welfare . . . (IPPF, 1980, 126–7)

This liberal attitude on one page seems, however, to be contradicted on the next. Wariness about too easily agreeing to the procedure is advised, with guidelines offered on the ways in which consultants and practitioners need to exercise caution in a number of areas. The legal framework of the country must be considered as well as the doctor's responsibility to the psychological and sociological state of the applicant. The doctor must consider the existing family and ages of any children, the stability of the marriage and also take account of cultural and religious differences, or exercise particular caution if the woman had recently delivered a child, or soon after an abortion. Finally, surgeons were reminded of their right not to engage in procedures which may offend their conscience. According to IPPF, therefore, even though individuals should have every opportunity to take control of their own fertility and reproductive capacity, getting through what emerges as a profusion of conditions intent on guiding and supporting may result in the doctor feeling encouraged to engage in subjective considerations and to make decisions based on assessments of the personal lives of applicants. This may support and even shelter the doctor from potential criticism but is not of much help to women who believe that it is they alone who must be the final judge of what is best for them.

Defending the decision

The study of available sterilization services (Allen, 1985) suggested that consultants and doctors may have inappropriate opinions about who should as well as who should not be sterilized, with decisions taken based, in part, on the impression given by the patient or applicant and which may be as much an issue of class as appearance or demeanour.[6] There are hints at attitudes which belie the tolerance and patience so often portrayed as part of the professional image, with consultants using terms such as 'the young and irresponsible' or accusing people of being turncoats if they change their lives and their minds and return for reversal.

> However objective and dispassionate a professional may be, it is nevertheless possible that strongly held beliefs may affect the way in which counselling or information or advice is given. Professionals are often the gatekeepers to access to services and, indeed, doctors are the gatekeepers to access to the procedures involved in

sterilization (and vasectomy and termination of pregnancy . . .)
(Allen, 1985, 220)

It may be that fifteen or twenty years ago doctors were held in awe and
there was less questioning of their analysis and professional judgement
than may be so in the present day (with what appears to be an increasing
trend by some dissatisfied patients towards considering litigation), but
some disquiet was expressed at the ease with which some women were
sterilized (Allen, 1985). It was clear from Allen's study that the very
strength and status of the professional allowed for personal opinion to
creep in to professional judgement: this was considered to be no bad thing
and an appropriate responsibility for medics. The following extract from
an interview with a consultant seems to demonstrate the diarists' oft-
voiced complaint that their own motives for refusing to be mothers were
always under scrutiny.[7] They commented frequently on the ways in
which they were made to feel that average and normal equals mother
whilst the motives of women who want and have children are not
questioned.

> It might be a slightly strange decision, to be sterilized. It is quite
> important to examine the motivation of someone who wants to do
> it [my question 'how, strange?']. Well, 'strange' being unusual, put
> it like that. Not wrong, not reprehensible, but different from an
> average person with average aims and desires. If someone doesn't
> want to do something which doesn't quite fit the normal expecta-
> tions of society then we perhaps have to ask, what is the
> motivation behind that? Is it a straightforward, perfectly legit-
> imate request, or is it a reaction to something else, or a defence? I
> mean there might be some other perfectly good methods of control
> without taking such a definite step. (Consultant A.)

The remainder of the interview did throw into sharp relief a very real
dilemma for GPs and consultants and one that clearly exercised him. He
was concerned that he did not do anything which would be a cause of
regret for women for, as he quite reasonably pointed out, 'even if the
incidence of sterilization for childfree women is as much as half a per
cent', this was still an extremely small number of women. The only
information that he had available to him and which informed his
decision-making was in applications from and interviews with women,

sterilized after having children, who later regretted their action and returned for reversal.

> Occasionally when I've refused it has been on the grounds of age. For example, for someone of 21 years it's less than halfway through their reproductive life. I may say to come back in one year's time, use other methods in the mean time. I think that's acceptable. Then if they do that and then return, they show determination – and there's some defence because someone could say to me 'Why on earth did you sterilize someone so young?'. (Consultant A.)

The dilemma here lies in the struggle faced by women in even getting as far as an interview with a consultant and the women in this study had little time for the arguments which presented a cautious response to what was, for them, a long-term source of frustration, rebuffs and refusals. The diversity of women's positive and negative experiences with doctors, and of the whole process from enquiring about to undergoing the operation, was perceived by many of them as an issue of medical power and control. They described the struggle as being one in which they made a personal decision about their own bodies and the way in which they planned to cope with fertility and reproduction, but then found that they would have to request and apply for their decision to be considered.

Some of the younger women described the attitude of the doctors who were dealing with their applications as patronizing and dismissive. This appeared to support other stories which are common gossip among women who describe how they sometimes perceive a condescending manner towards them by some professionals in the medical world, particularly during pregnancy and childbirth, and if they are in need of any type of gynaecological treatment. Women's anecdotes tell of doctors speaking about rather than to them, and of questions and discussions between doctors, students and nurses being held across their body during physical examinations. The internal hierarchy of the medical profession does not encourage challenges and disagreements, particularly at consultant level, and it is likely to be here that many childfree women seeking sterilization find the greatest area of conflict and experience the power of final refusal.

The role of doctor – particularly GP – is one based on the reasonable assumption that patients are unwell in some way and expect to be made better: the relationship is one of healer and to-be-healed, with the doctor prescribing medicines or other treatments to that end. Yet, a request made for elective sterilization, based on an individual's decision rather than expert medical diagnosis, challenges these expected and commonly adopted roles of doctor and patient. Women who are otherwise well and visit their doctor to request not healing, nor medication nor expert advice, but an operation which, in medical terms, is non-essential, seem to be using the doctor primarily as a means to an end. Rather than the usual procedure of a GP making a referral after examination and diagnosis, doctors may feel that their particular level of professionalism is useful for the applicant only for her to gain access to the next stage in the process, an interview with a consultant.

Doctors have a wealth of expertise based on experience and practice and considerable professional authority vested in their status and the role of medical practitioner. There is little immediate opportunity for a patient who disagrees with a diagnosis or judgement to demand that it is reconsidered or overturned, often because the doctor will present authoritative reasons for having reached the particular conclusion. The diarists' reports of 'being laughed out of the surgery', and their feelings of being helpless in the face of such authority and 'not being taken seriously' are negative examples of the power relationship between doctor and patient and confirmed for some that they would need to seek sterilization elsewhere, usually through paying for private consultation or with BPAS and Marie Stopes's centres. Some doctors' reasoning suggested that they suspected an underlying agenda for a request which they felt justified in viewing with caution: Consultant A.'s response seemed to illustrate this doubt when he queried whether or not a request was 'straightforward and perfectly legitimate, a reaction to something else, or a defence?'.

This suspicion was not confined to medical practitioners but also appeared as a feature of other professions involved with women's reproduction. Some counsellors found people who were adamant in their views very difficult to counsel, especially if they were young, using subjective language and expressing opinions and assessments which seemed to be based on their own reactions in feeling the need to understand and make sense of the determination of the applicants. There appeared to be strong counter-argument and attempts at dissuasion in some of the encounters and an element of 'infantizing' and occasional refusal to accept the validity of the case and reasons presented for sterilization. Isobel Allen's interviews highlighted some of these views and the following selection illustrates what applicants may have experienced as resistance to their application.

'I point out that to deal with a headache you don't have to cut your head off'; 'I have an idea that the group of people who never want children have had unhappy childhoods'; '[it was] difficult to counsel people who were absolutely insistent that they want to be sterilized, often when very young and for idealistic reasons'; 'I suspect that there are times when you get involved. I did say to one girl of 19 that she was totally wrong. She wanted to be sterilized because of world overpopulation. I said she could see the doctor. He wasn't happy either . . . '. (extracts from interviews, in Allen, 1985, 250–1)

Refusal or attempts to dissuade mainly concentrated on sterilization applications from women and there was an indication that 'professionals' concern' may have been used to influence the outcome of meetings with women who were determined to continue applying for sterilization. Whilst professionals have equal power of refusal over men and women this may be wielded unevenly, with women being treated in a more paternalistic way because it was thought that men could be better relied upon to know their own minds (Allen, 1985). Many of the diarists emphasized their belief that it is they, more than many other women, who give more than a passing thought to this major life decision which will affect not only themselves and those near to them, but also the very life of the newborn.

Responsibility – that is why I don't want children . . . there are children all over the world starving, abused and neglected, chil-dren who have been created and moulded by sadness, despair and survive in the face of abhorrent situations and dangerous adults. I couldn't have a child and add to that pain, the overcrowding of the world, not when there are human beings out there who exist alone. To add to the problem is to ignore our responsibility to stop and change it. (Emma)

There were strong reactions to any suggestion that their decision, in this most deeply personal part of their lives, was open to question and criticism or that they could be called to account for making a decision which, in their opinion, was well considered and thoroughly explored, and they felt that most women who have children do not usually engage in such extensive considerations and decision-making. Vicky stressed that women should think more carefully about the pressures that having children bring: 'after reading Jane Bartlett's book *Will You Be Mother?* I agreed with the women who recognized in themselves an incipient baby-batterer. I loathe mess and noise and people continually craving my attention – even my cats rarely get stroked!' The reason sometimes given for children being an essential part of family life did not hold up for Sandy. She rejected the suggestion from friends about regretting her decision and being lonely in old age; 'people who have children just to fill their old age with grandchildren will be sadly let down.'

A critical self-awareness of personal abilities and aptitudes came through in several interviews and Sally was overwhelmed with the thought of having to be responsible for another life and did not feel confident that she could do it. She saw herself as being part of a society in which all adults have responsibilities to look after the children and to care for them, 'but I didn't want one for myself. When people used to ask me whether I had children when I was 21 or so, I used to think, but I'm just a child myself!'. Gemma's scribbled postscript on an otherwise quite sober and formal letter to the consultant prior to her interview was painfully honest: 'I'm not patient, tolerant, calm or practical enough to cope. I doubt I'd have the energy and I don't like "suffering" in others, nor doing things when I feel incompetent'. The sense of power and control that adults are able to exert over a vulnerable child was viewed with unease by some diarists who included such feelings in their rationale for deciding not to have children:

> I think people like myself who have been sterilized before having children have given far more thought to that than women who do have children. In the same way that people say 'I want a child', I say 'I don't want a child'. I often think what could be more selfish than saying 'I want a child'? It's a big ego trip having a child, don't you think? You create a person and instil your own ideas of right and wrong and moral values. (Linda L.)

The diarists presented a firm commitment to their strongly held rationale for having made the choice to remain childfree (if, indeed, they considered that they had made a choice).[8] As most of the women knew no one else like themselves, and as they appeared to have arrived at their conviction having discussed it with very few others – usually close family members and intimate friends – the role of counselling, in the early stage of the process of choosing to have no children and as part of the medical interviews, appeared to play little or no part for the women in making the decision to be sterilized.

Counselling for sterilization

Sterilization performed for anything other than medical reasons dates only from the late 1960s after various legislative abortion reforms: counselling for the procedure, therefore, is as yet in its early stages. The provision of counselling services in this area of life-defining decisions is patchy or negligible and what is available – usually within the medical model – concentrates mainly on checking the determination of the applicant by dint of the 'what if?' questions, attempting to persuade individuals to try another form of contraception or providing practical information about the details of the operation once the procedure had been agreed. These otherwise essential elements do not address the fundamental purpose of counselling, which is to provide a supportive context within which, amongst other things, individuals have the space and time to explore and examine their personal motivation, choices and decisions and, if appropriate, as a way of resolving their unique questions.[9]

Because being childfree is an area which has attracted much adverse and critical comment, it may be assumed that many of the childfree women interviewed had experienced a modicum of uncertainty and even emotional struggle in attempting to weigh and balance both sides of an argument and consider the pros and cons of having children. Questions asked at interview and requests for such reflections to be included in diaries were intended to allow the opportunity for women to relate any problems encountered and their ways of overcoming them so as to find ways through the complexities and the barriers of the medical world. It was also, by being able to draw on memories of their early childfree choice and the later decision to be sterilized, to provide space to describe any feelings of isolation or where they judged it appropriate to remain stoic, controlled and silent.[10] This line of questioning was based on the assumption that the women who responded to the advertisement for participants in the study had wanted, but were unlikely to have found, the type of counselling services which would have supported and validated their choice. Not only was this not the case, but also (as evinced by Geraldine's comment that she viewed counselling as yet one more stalling tactic) most of the women displayed a disregard of initiating anything which involved them in having to explore an issue about which they had, for the most part, 'always known'.

An extensive study of counselling for abortion and sterilization procedures showed that 93 per cent of professionals said that they provided either counselling or opportunities for discussion (Allen, 1985). During interviews for this study with medical practitioners and family planning advisers, it emerged that the terminology and the way that the word 'counselling' was being used was significantly adrift. The meaning given to counselling (as used by the women as well as medical professionals) highlighted that it was intended to provide advice and information about the practical aspects of the operation and aftermath rather than allowing an opportunity to explore personal questions and emotional uncertainties. The practicalities are undoubtedly essential, but appeared to be concerned only with confirming that the decision made by the applicant was secure, and that the medical procedure was explored and appreciated. This was an aspect which worried some who were involved in the process and who expressed a wish that counselling should cover feelings as well as giving information. Often the line of questioning about the firmness of the decision was felt to be irrelevant and could include asking how the applicant would feel if their children died or if the current relationship ended. Such questions can easily be dismissed and allow a mechanical response mainly because they are far too hypothetical and beyond people's expectations of their current realities (Allen 1985).

Far from experiencing early life uncertainties, the greatest problem for the childfree women diarists was identified again and again as other people's reactions, and how to cope with that. Many of the women had used their network of family and friends for personal support and guidance in exploring the issues. It may be inferred that, for them, this was the counselling element, although not every woman could, nor even would, consider discussing their personal issues with people so close. Most of the women were satisfied with the level, style and content of the counselling that they received but some wondered whether it would suit every woman. Anne D. felt that the counsellor provided by the Marie Stopes clinic she attended was 'so glib, really, it took 5 minutes. I didn't mind as I was sure, but it made me wonder for those who needed more.'

Women who use the BPAS or other of the family planning services rather than only the GP would have their concerns recognized and sympathetically dealt with even if only for a short time, probably a maximum of three sessions, yet although both medical information and counselling and advice are seen by BPAS teams as being equally essential, long-term counselling is not on offer. Within the health and medical services there is not a tradition or facility for counselling for medical conditions; 'just as we don't counsel for most other areas of women's health, we don't counsel for sterilization' (Consultant B.).

In all of the discussions and descriptions given by the diarists about any counselling, only Jane gave a personal account of what was clearly a defining moment in a positive and worthwhile experience. She had continued using contraception during the many years when she wavered in her decision-making about motherhood and, in this regard, she appears to exemplify Carolyn Morrell's 'postponer' description of women who felt sterilization to be 'too final'. Jane's decision to have a child was confirmed and consolidated at a meeting with her counsellor;

> I described my feelings with the counsellor and said I wanted to be able to sort out my feelings so I could make my decision, and she listened and then just looked at me. Then she said, 'But you know what you want to do, don't you?' and straight away I said 'Yes, I do – I really want a child'. As I drove away I just thought it was as if I was a big 'YES'. It was like my whole body was saying 'YES'. (Jane)

The study of counselling services for sterilization and vasectomy (Allen, 1985) appeared to confirm a lack of counselling provision, but this was matched by a seeming lack of demand. It was acknowledged that there are some people who do need access to the type of counselling which will support them in making their own appropriate decision: it seems that others do not.

> It was quite clear from interviews with consumers that there were people who needed very little counselling, whose circumstances were such that they had come to an informed decision after considerable discussion with their partners, friends and relations, having tried all contraceptive methods, and having decided that,

for them, sterilization . . . was what they wanted. (Allen, 1985, 246)

The provision currently available within the medical services seldom allows for the complex processing that women undertake which leads to their opting for sterilization. The diarists and women in other studies appeared to be cautious about expressing anything other than absolute determination as they sensed that anything less could signal uncertainty which, they feared, would lead to certain refusal. None the less, for those women who may feel the need to explore any and every aspect of this enormously significant life decision, the provision of counselling services of some kind and of however limited a duration could provide opportunities for childfree women to have maximum opportunity to examine thoroughly their motivation and decision. Such a service may also go some way to allaying the necessary fears of doctors and consultants when faced with a childfree woman intent on elective sterilization.

Notes

1. The issue of people using sarcasm towards those who have no children by making reference to cats and other pets as 'child substitutes' was raised so often that it now seems to border on 'urban myth'. Jacky Fleming's cartoon of a woman stroking a cat and asking 'Is this your substitute for children?' elicits the response from a fed-up-looking young woman: 'No. It's a domestic cat'. Carolyn Morell remarks on 'compensatory ideology', which she describes as the 'prevalent cultural view . . . that among the childless, attachments to animals signify a substitution for the missing child' (Morell, 1994, 90). One would imagine from these comments that there are no pets in homes with children, and that Britain's 'nation of dog-lovers' consists entirely of childfree women.
2. Freud asserted that 'Anatomy is destiny' and at the heart of his theory of sexual difference is the visibility of difference: the anatomically 'correct' male, complete with penis compared with the absence of this visible sexual organ from the body of woman. Arising from this was his assertion that the girl child's lack of a penis leads her to penis envy, and that her subsequent need for children (and even her intellectual and career needs) is determined by the need to substitute for the penis which she so desires:

   > At no other point in one's analytic work does one suffer more from an oppressive feeling that all one's repeated efforts have been in vain – than when one is trying to persuade a woman to abandon her wish for a penis on the grounds of its being unrealizable. (Freud, 1937, in Mitchell and Rose, 1982, 7)

3. The choice of a word to describe and give a name to women without children taxed me for a time, but my decision to use childfree was based on my own long-term use

of the word and acknowledgement of its meanings for me. It is recognized in Britain and America and for a short time I read contributions to the well-subscribed American Net-list 'child-free', which possibly provides there what BON (British Organisation for Non-Parents) provides in the UK. Carolyn Morell dislikes childfree:

> childless by choice. The phrase itself signifies lack . . . this term (childfree) has a presumptuous ring to it. It suggests that women who do not have children of their own want to be rid of children, as in those who promote a 'union-free' or 'smoke-free' environment'. (Morell, 1994, 21)

The lack of a term for women choosing to remain without children reinforces what she goes on to describe as 'the dominant ideology which views mother as superior'. My use of the word, both written and spoken, was neither queried nor commented on by the women in this study, and they used the same term to me in interview and during discussion.

4. This was the major motivation in my own application for sterilization at the age of 32.
5. During my interviews with several consultants and family planning advisers, I asked whether they used such a rule or if they considered that it would be useful: although some had heard of it, the rule did not seem to be a guiding principle for decisions. Jane Bartlett comments in passing on this rule (Bartlett, 1994, 144–6).
6. Allen's study in 1985 identified the probable class differentials of sterilization being suggested by doctors, or of women reaching such a decision for themselves.
7. Sally insisted that she had never considered becoming a mother nor did she make an active decision not to have a child, nor positively choose to be childfree.
8. There were many comments – some angry and others astonished or bemused – and references to occasions when the childfree decision was attacked and vilified, whereas when a pregnancy was announced there was usually fulsome praise and congratulations for the mother-to-be.
9. The interpretation of counselling is based on the definition and guidelines of the British Association for Counselling, with its proposition that 'the skilled and principled use of relationship' is central to facilitating and developing 'self-knowledge, emotional acceptance and growth and . . . personal resources'. This relationship concentrates on the needs of the client, focused on 'resolving specific problems [and] working through feelings of inner conflict'. (BAC, 1995).
10. An interesting parallel may be drawn with childfree women and involuntarily childless women in that when the latter seek infertility treatment they feel that it is essential not to show any ambivalence in their desire for having a child in case their application is viewed less favourably. Sterilization applicants also resolved to present a complete determination so that their applications would not be jeopardized because of their being seen as uncertain or a 'waverer'. I am indebted to Gayle Letherby for her insights and comments on this.

5

Sterilization as a Positive Choice

Seeing women as 'childless by choice' may be accurate at a simple descriptive level. But it misplaces the emphasis and misstates what was chosen. Women are expected to explain a negative occurrence, a negative choice. The absence of motherhood becomes the point of focus rather than the many prior positive choices. (Morell, 1994, 50)

There was an expression by the women, in both their diaries and during interviews, of their overwhelming relief at having made a significant transition. Each one felt that she had moved from being a woman who had chosen not to have children but who, in theory, continued to be capable of doing so, to being a woman who had decided to be sterilized and, therefore, would never have children. In various ways they described having no regrets about making their decision and their determination to pursue sterilization even in the face of persistent rebuttal of their arguments and refusal of their applications.

Jude's response typified much of the rationale and many of the sentiments expressed by most diarists when she described the inadequacy of available contraception and feelings of being unwilling any longer to live with the potential damage to her body: 'so, for me, sterilization was a natural progression from unsatisfactory contraception'.

> My first request for sterilization resulted in me being laughed out of the surgery by the male GP. Later, when I went to see my woman GP she was obviously surprised but respectful and she contacted a gynaecologist at my local hospital. I spent a long time getting my arguments and reasons ready as I expected to have to put my case very strongly and have to persuade the consultant. I had hardly begun my argument when he just said 'That's fine, you've obviously thought it through'. He asked me 'What if at thirty-five the urge hits?' and I said 'Well, I would adopt' but then I felt angry and disappointed with myself. I wanted to get him off my back, I knew that I definitely never wanted children, wouldn't adopt, but I was aware all the time that he had the power to refuse. I was frightened that my response wasn't good enough and I just kept thinking 'Oh, God, don't take this away from me now . . .'.
> (Jude)

When preparing to present their case for sterilization most of the women said that they felt the need to construct an acceptable story and reported feeling wary and under pressure to present what 'they' – that is, the GPs and consultants – wanted to hear. Some women had been coached by other women who advised that the doctor or consultant would be likely to probe personal details and might ask about future possibilities (they described these as the 'what if . . . ?' questions) but that these were standard and it was probably best to accept passively what was said, to have rehearsed answers ready but definitely to hold back on true feelings. It was also important to be aware that there could be challenging questions and Anne T. had been pre-warned by a friend that the male consultant would probably ask what would be her response if a knight on a white charger appeared; 'I just told him that I didn't believe in fairy stories!'. Jude was terrified that her argument was not good enough and echoes other statements and comments about women feeling the need to tread cautiously and be careful about how they responded. This often ended in their feeling compromised and unable to be fully truthful.

The fine – and often invisible – line between being assertive and determined needed to be recognized and negotiated. The women had to be convincing and certain of their ground but remain sufficiently calm and restrained so as not to antagonize the one person who held the power to refuse, thus scuppering the latest chance. Like Anne T., Vicky had had some advice about when to keep quiet and when to appear firm and determined;

> I was schooled, I suppose, for the interview by the consultant's secretary (we had worked together) and she said to keep firmly in mind what he wanted to hear, that if he refused me a sterilization and I did get pregnant I must say that I would be coming back to him for an abortion. (Vicky)

This part of the story-telling to doctors appeared as being an essential element for women in overcoming any reluctance that they encountered. They felt that if there was a balance of decision being made, many doctors might be persuaded by reference to a determination for undergoing abortions in future. This was not always successful, however, especially in the often long chain of various medical contexts in which women found themselves.

> My GP was totally supportive of my decision having known me since my teens. The gynaecologist was less so and I ended up telling him I would have an abortion if I ever became pregnant (I had been told that this was the thing to say). He pointed out that one woman in ten who comes for the op. changes their minds (meaning that nine in ten don't!). He basically acted as 'devil's advocate' and tried his best to dissuade me despite my arguments. Eventually he agreed but said he would put me on a waiting list and it would be a year's wait. After two years a different consultant could see that I was totally adamant and was helpful in moving me up the list. (Sandy)

Women who apply for sterilization seem to be in no doubt of their feeling that GPs and consultants will make them 'jump through hoops'. Somehow this seemed to be viewed by both sides as a necessary part of the procedure although, inevitably, it appeared to the applicants that the power lay on one side only. The nurse at a family planning centre was certain that women have to 'pass a test', usually in the form of a 'cat-and-mouse' question and answer procedure. She was aware that the waiting room at the centre was a place where women could exchange information and advise others on the best way to go about getting what they wanted:

they think, 'If I say the right thing then I'll get what I want', and to each other, 'Well, you have to say this, that and the other and then she'll say yes'. I don't want women to feel like that – they should feel it's more open and discussed. (Nurse specialist)

As well as the anxieties expressed about what they felt was an already assumed agenda for their meetings with doctors and consultants, the diarists were also uncomfortably aware of the reticence expressed by those in the medical world about women's motivations for sterilization. Some were puzzled and, like Linda L., even angrily questioned the motivations of men in entering an exclusively female world.

I don't know any women gynaecologists. Are there any? It's always intrigued me that men want to be gyny's. They say God's a man, and then when a man gets to be a gynaecologist they can really pretend they are! (Linda L.)

Being sterilized

After reflecting on and describing the often frustrating, infuriating and occasionally humiliating journeys leading to having their application for sterilization accepted, the women in this study made much less of the operation itself. They identified the hospital or service used and whether they had had to pay, yet there were few details given about the procedure other than the method (clips, ties or cauterization).

I finally had my operation at 40. I didn't have any choice of method but I was so relieved to find someone who would do the operation without any qualms and on the NHS that he could have used a stapler, string or any other method – I didn't care. I could have kissed him! (Pauline)

In describing their individual recollections, the most commented on aspect was of relief at being taken seriously and knowing that their personal birth control was resolved. There was an occasional, sometimes almost casual, remark about pain or discomfort, and both Ginny and Linda R. had a few uncomfortable days as a result of the gas used during the operation procedure, experiencing shoulder ache and feeling blown-up with wind. This meant wearing the only clothing that felt comfortable, and for Linda R. that was a tent-shaped Indian cotton dress. Jill's memory was her positive feelings at being on first-name terms with the surgeon and being able to choose a general anaesthetic so that 'the actual op. was quite a good experience. I was euphoric when I came round and felt a huge relief'. The discomfort experienced by Gemma was then followed by fear, as she had some unexpected bleeding and, lacking basic aftercare information, needed to telephone the hospital ward to check on whether she should take 'any special action'. There were no complications with the small incisions and, despite her stomach feeling 'vulnerable' for the first week, 'I've been able to forget all about it – so to speak!'.

Feeling that she was in control was essential for Linda L. and she stressed that, for her, paying for the operation ensured that she was able to say exactly what she wanted and when.

> I wanted to have it done privately as I couldn't justify using the NHS for something I personally wanted. I felt that I might be cheating someone who might have needed a life-threatening operation. I wanted to have it done for my own 'selfish' reasons. Because I was paying I had complete control. I chose just before Easter so as not to use up my holiday time and I could rest up. Generally the whole experience was very positive and everyone was very helpful. The medical staff really looked after me. (Linda L.)

A few diarists commented on the ways in which other medical staff, such as nurses and even hospital orderlies, behaved towards them. Judith found the people in the medical profession to be helpful 'in a detached kind of way' and Sally's assessment of the treatment that she had received was that it had been excellent, but she followed it with the remark that 'at no time was I treated as or made to feel odd'. Some diarists seemed to be particularly sensitive about the nature of their operation, although it is possible that their feelings of isolation in their choice and action enhanced this and there were criticisms, such as those made by Judith of the seeming insensitivity of being placed in hospital wards with women who were undergoing treatment for infertility, or other gynaecological procedures, and even with women who had suffered miscarriages and stillbirths of their babies.

For some of the women, being sterilized for contraceptive purposes solved only half of their problem and they welcomed further surgery.

When further gynaecological problems emerged necessitating hysterectomy, not all of the diarists found this to be a totally negative experience. Gillian found that she was left with some dysfunctional bleeding problems resulting in her undergoing a hysterectomy in 1984, whilst Jean described her operation as very straightforward and then 'last year I had a hysterectomy and this was the best feature of all – no more periods!!'. However, not all of the sterilization operations were fully successful and several women recounted experiences which appeared to be painful and inconvenient and, for some, traumatic and potentially life-threatening.

> The only difficulty was that between the GP and the consultant appointments I had salpingitis and the 'sterilization consultant' diagnosed fibroids. I was admitted for a hysterectomy but, in fact, had an ovarian cyst removed and had the tubes tied at the same time. So there were lots of operation after-effects which were not really connected with sterilization. (Anne T.)

Despite Jill's feeling of euphoria immediately after the operation, she continued to bleed heavily each month, which she suffered for a further thirteen years until it was discovered that the surgeon had failed to remove her IUD, as requested during the sterilization procedure. She wrote that 'I suppose it was due to an administrative or medical error. Fortunately no permanent damage was done, just thirteen years of heavy bleeding – now blissfully ended.' In comparison with vasectomy, the method used for male sterilization, tubal ligation does have known hazards and side effects and is fraught with complications which threaten the health of many women (Turner, 1993). According to family planning organization figures, it is estimated tht more than 150 million women throughout the world 'are protected by sterilisation' (Marie Stopes International, publicity material, June 1995): globally this makes laparoscopic sterilization the single most common method of controlling fertility. Whereas, for most of the women in this study, the operation was reported as having few long-term effects, the aftermath of the procedure was much more serious and traumatic for Geraldine.

> I would like to tell you that everything is fine, that I've no regrets and am living happily ever after, but I can't. Four years after the sterilization I had an ectopic pregnancy which almost cost me my life then an ovarian cyst and further surgery, and a total hysterectomy six months after that. Apparently ectopics are common after

sterilization but nobody warned me about that. Sterilization did, without doubt, give me a lot of unplanned experiences! (Geraldine)

After sterilization: relief and regret

The caution expressed by practitioners in the medical profession about the inevitability of women's future regrets about the finality of their lost fertility were not echoed in the interviews with the women diarists. Indeed, the opposite was the case. The overwhelming feeling portrayed was of relief at having the necessity removed of continuing to take contraception. Several women emphasized that, because they had reached their decision about being childfree far in advance of considering sterilization, it was the freedom from the fear of being let down by contraceptive methods that was at the forefront of thinking: it was not the chance to change their minds or the lost opportunity for a baby.

The most frequently asked questions which women encountered whilst waiting for their applications to be considered related to the alternatives to surgery: 'Why choose sterilization as the means of ensuring against pregnancy and motherhood?'; 'Why not stay with the methods of contra- ception you have used so far?'; or 'When you reach your thirties or forties, how do you know that you won't regret being unable to have babies and then apply for a reversal?'. These type of questions were often asked, not only by those who are genuinely puzzled by a childfree lifestyle, but also by doctors and consultants to whom applications for sterilization are made. Childfree women felt that they were well able to give answers to all of those queries but complained that their reasons were considered insufficient, in part because of the general resistance to sterilizing childfree women. They are not seen as having distinctly differ- ent motivations from the many women who have had children and then, believing that they have completed their family, opt for sterilization in order to give up using contraception: for diverse reasons, some women with children do later apply for reversal in order to have more children.

As yet there is no national up-to-date breakdown of the annual figures for sterilized women who later have the procedure reversed and yet doctors and consultants appear to reach a decision to refuse applications for sterilization from childfree women on the basis that most women will regret making the decision and will return for reversal at a future period in their lives. The women in this study were very familiar with – and frustrated by – this argument.

> When the present serious relationship began I knew I didn't want to go back on the Pill. I asked about contraception and steriliza-tion but the doctor felt that I'd only recently been widowed and there was every possibility I'd change my mind. He said that most women come asking for sterilization then come back a couple of years later saying they wanted babies, but this is women who've had children. I'm sure that he said that because I was a woman with no children. (Linda L.)

Most childfree women in this study said that at some point in the time leading to their sterilization a comment had been made about future regrets and reversals. There are indications that sterilization as a method of contraception is becoming more popular, but there is also an increase in requests for reversal (Allen, 1985), with almost two-thirds of the professionals involved in the area of fertility contraception and birth control reporting that a new partner or other changes in life circum-stances were the main reasons cited by people who apply for reversal. Rather than attempting to convince her questioner that she would never change her mind, Sally tackled the issue head on;

> I do remember one question which was 'Do you think you might change your mind in future?' I assured her that, like most normal people I had no idea! I did know, however, that my experience told me that I am able to live with taking wrong decisions and I don't think I would ever regret a decision I had taken as long as it had been taken freely and with all the facts. (Sally)

The counselling and written information available to applicants for sterilization makes clear and always stresses that it should be considered as permanent, yet an interesting twist to this emerged in a study con-ducted in the mid-1970s by Professor Lord Robert Winston, a specialist who is currently an eminent consultant in the field of infertility. His examination of the reasons given by 103 women requesting reversals showed that the most common were remarriage, a new partnership and wanting a child in that partnership. The study noted

> [that some people asked for reversal] knowing that there was perhaps only a slim chance of its being successful, but in order to

show their new partner that they had 'tried'. It was regarded in some way as a commitment. (Winston, 1977, in Allen, 1985, 253)[1]

Undoubtedly the requests for reversal are genuine in that, if successful, the new partnership may produce a child as intended, but this reasoning is characteristic of people who are already parents and not of women who say categorically that they have never wanted to have children. Despite the concerns about these people, felt by a number of doctors who are convinced that there will be later regrets, some consultants affirmed that these were often the very people who never regretted it or asked for reversals and they would still persevere with their requests even if they were refused or told to wait for a while and to reconsider what they were asking (Allen, 1985).

The diarists identified that two years seemed to be a standard period of doctors using 'delay-time', and what they considered to be concerted attempts to put off the request for as long as possible is supported in a paper by a leading specialist in the field (Newton, 1982). In his survey of four studies on the changing patterns of male and female sterilization, he identified the difficulties encountered by 38 childfree women in obtaining an NHS sterilization. They had held firm views on what they wanted for many years but had been 'fobbed off' with remarks like 'wait a little' or 'you're too young'. As Sandy's story appears to show, doctors may indeed be aware that women in general are unlikely to regret sterilization, as the gynaecologist who conducted the consultation with her focused on the one in ten women who do return for reversal rather than the nine in ten who do not.

Isobel Allen's major study of the availability of services for counselling, sterilization and vasectomy (Allen, 1985) provided detailed information on significant aspects of sterilization and of the women who undergo the operation but the study also made clear that, although sterilization reversals requests had increased, it was virtually impossible to make an entirely accurate estimate of the annual incidence of female sterilization, nor was it possible to be clear about the numbers of requests for reversal. However, a leading specialist provided the answer to a question on this and his reply confirmed what was being strongly signalled throughout this study: that sterilization is recorded only by a male or female break-down, and no national collation of the reasons for requests and applications are readily available. The same consultant also responded to my enquiry about requests for reversals from sterilized childfree women and his reply indicated that there are very few childfree women who return for reversal and yet they are considered to be no different from women who have had children and who do return and say that they regret having had the operation.

> I would say that of the 700 sterilizations that I have reversed, in the order of 20 of these were women who had been sterilized without ever having had any children, because they believed that they would never want to have a family. Of the rest, the great majority believe that they have completed child bearing having had one or more child. (Professor Lord Robert Winston, letter, 13 Dec. 1996)

A similar response to the question was voiced at interview by both of the consultant gynaecologists, with Consultant A. saying that approximately ten childfree women had applied for sterilization during his fourteen years at the hospital and 'I couldn't say how many women without children apply for reversal, but I'd hazard very few'. Consultant B. also confirmed the very small numbers concerned:

> I really couldn't say what are the figures for reversal although I'm sure it's right that very few return. Once these women have fought their way through and got what they want because of the premiss on which they want to run their lives they would not be the sort of people who would want it reversed, whatever happens. (Consultant B.)

On a few occasions the childfree women in this study spoke angrily about women who are mothers applying for sterilization reversal: they felt that it was because of such apparently fickle behaviour that they were cast in the same mould. This appears to be a dualistic perception which results in a polarization of women into categories of either rational or irrational. This simple way of dividing women may allow them to be more easily dealt with by the medical gatekeepers and could lead to the type of behaviour towards them which, in their diaries and during interviews, the diarists described as patronizing, infantizing and dismissive. There was some annoyance expressed around this issue, though more often rather a feeling of indignation at being so misunderstood; 'those of us who decide to be sterilized don't change our minds or regret what we've chosen. I have never had a single regret, and as a bonus my sex life improved dramatically after the operation!' (Jill).

To some of those holding power in the medical profession, a woman reversing her previously strongly held conviction that she would remain childfree represents – even proves – fickleness, or indecision or evidence of her inability to know her own mind. However, the woman's own perception may be that such a change is a progressive feature of her life experiences and part of her individual personal development. Similarly, a change of heart and reasons for regret happen to some women who have had children, despite the careful prior consideration they gave to the decision to be sterilized; a decision likely to have been based mainly on reaching the point where they believed their families to be complete. However, over the course of their life they have experiences which could not have been predicted and which impact on previous strongly held convictions and prior actions (Allen, 1985).

Women sterilized after having children have experienced what it is like to be a parent and, because of the many genuine reasons which prompt a change of mind, including the commitment to a new relationship, they may desire to have more children with a partner and so request a reversal. At the point at which both women who are mothers and childfree women decide to apply for sterilization they share a major identical reason for doing so. They all want to avoid accidental pregnancy and unplanned children with the additional bonus of no longer needing to use contraception.

With one exception all of the childfree women in this study made it clear that they felt that they had made a positive choice, that having children held no allure and that they had made strenuous efforts to avoid the state of motherhood. Heather is the only one out of the diarists who has come to regret her sterilization – although she had been very sure and positive about her original decision – and had applied for reversal after she and her husband took over the care of her nephew, the baby son of her sister who died tragically young. She wrote movingly about this in her diary under the heading 'A Change of Heart' (a further extract from Heather's diary is included in the Appendix).

My sister was diagnosed with a rare type of cancer and was subsequently unable to look after her two young sons so J. and I took [the baby of thirteen months] most weekends and holidays. This was a revelation – in practical terms, that I could do it! – but also emotionally. I had endless patience with him, I was fiercely protective and I could understand and relate to him. I found that these experiences were slowly but surely changing my mind about motherhood. Well, I ENJOYED him, even whilst not daring to think of him as 'our little boy'. My relationship with J. reached new depths and with it the desire to have a child of our own. I felt that we had a lot to give and that parenthood would enrich our own lives. I went back and asked if a reversal would be possible. After much soul-searching, considering the long wait, possible failure, my age and the possibility of a Down's Syndrome child we decided not to go ahead . . . Meanwhile I live with a decision that can be counted as the ONLY regret that I hold in an otherwise very happy and fulfilling life. (Heather)

This account of Heather's reasons for applying for reversal, and the sorrowful experience of bereavement followed closely by her moving description of discovering the potential to love a child, bear out Allen's findings that professionals found that there was 'no magic formula for preventing regrets' and for dealing with women's personal choices and decisions about their own reproduction and fertility. The study concluded that people must be given all of the facts that they requested and cautioned not to make hasty decisions early in their lives and especially not during or after any stressful time. There must be great emphasis on the procedure being considered as irreversible but, nevertheless, people must be allowed to take final responsibility for their own lives, especially as the type and manner of changes of circumstances which might lead to future regrets and reversal requests are usually impossible to foresee (Allen, 1985).

The disapproving and negative manner in which medics view reversals for childfree women highlights that there is also a clearly discriminatory aspect to applications for sterilization, with women being afforded differential treatment on the basis of their status as 'mother'. Regardless of the struggle undertaken by childfree women to reach a consultant, in most instances they will not be considered to have a serious case and so they will be infantized and told to continue with other forms of contraception. This instruction will be based on the unresearched and unsubstantiated opinion that childfree women will later regret being sterilized and return for reversal. Currently, whatever data exists refers specifically to women with children: childfree women who elect for sterilization or reversal remain unidentified or unrecorded as such.

Once safely through the hazardous and chancy period whereby their every motive and emotion was scrutinized for some hint that they were not fully committed, a few diarists felt able to explore their feelings about motherhood and how it could have been for them to have become mothers. Most of the women said that it was essential to express a rigid determination in the face of what they experienced as often hostile questioning which appeared to test for any hint of uncertainty or potential future regret. In this way, it could be that they were acknowledging the importance and necessity of presenting a more determined front than perhaps was necessary. Pauline wrote that, although she was greatly relieved to be sterilized and never regretted her decision, she sometimes did wonder what motherhood might have been like and Judith expanded on the attendant ambivalences;

> Regrets? Of course, sometimes . . . but not for long and they are pure emotion rather than rational! I'm not a person who spends much time looking back. Once a decision is made I go forward and get on with whatever the consequences are. I did get occasional pangs of wistfulness, having had a negative experience of pregnancy as a teenager and having to keep it secret. I sometimes thought it would be good to have a pregnancy to be proud of . . . but it was a dream, really! (Judith)

Far from being an eagerly awaited and welcomed state, childfree women perceive motherhood in negative terms; for them, the affirmative practice is to remain without children (Morell, 1994). Most of the childfree sterilized women in this study acknowledged early on in their lives that motherhood had no appeal, preferring to explore what for them were the many contemporary attractive, desirable and realizable alternatives to becoming a mother. By making active choices regarding contraceptive measures, they ensured that they were able to maintain their childfree status and lifestyles. Having done so, and despite the hostility shown to the childfree decision and an assumption that it was a negative choice, they were firm in their belief that remaining childfree and deciding to be sterilized were based on positive decisions about their futures. They felt that the gratifications of their present life would be compromised by having children and there was also the danger of missing out on unknown future opportunities and possibilities. For these women it was having children that was problematic – an attitude which upends traditional beliefs and expectations that women only have positive maternal feelings and are willingly prepared to give up parts of their lives for the unknown and untried advantages to be gained through entering the state of motherhood.

Note

1. As part of a new relationship, my childfree partner and I discussed the possibility of a reversal of my sterilization. After further consideration and a meeting with a consultant, we decided that we would continue as a couple without attempting to have children. I recognized my past situation instantly when I read the observant conclusion by Professor Winston that, in new partnerships where one or both of the couple has children and one is sterilized so preventing their having a child together, just such 'a commitment' may be part of the early stages of confirming and bonding the relationship.

Reflections on a process – Jude, April 1997

When I first saw the advert in *Everywoman* my initial feeling was one of relief. At that time I was feeling not only that I was the 'only one' but that having a sterilization in order to remain childfree was a taboo issue and one that was not being discussed or covered in any area. I felt reassured immediately, and validated that a feminist researcher was doing this work. It took away the sense of isolation and the feeling of being a freak!

I waited with great anticipation to hear from Annily and looking back I realize that was about my need to somehow connect with other women in my position, and a need to talk through the process with another feminist working on this issue. As a feminist activist I also felt a sense of urgency to discuss my experience and what it meant politically.

I received the questionnaire soon after and remember the process of responding to the questions as very significant. I wrote over fifteen pages, and could have written more. It was incredibly important and affirming writing down not only why I had taken the decision and what it was like to have it, but it was crucial for me to share, with Annily and other childfree women (and I felt that I was sharing with them even though we had had no direct contact as yet), the responses I had had to what I had done, and to hear their experiences too. But most importantly as an activist I needed to reflect upon and say what it meant politically about women's position in society and state that clearly to the world – this book is doing that for me, like a form of fighting back.

I believe the process of being interviewed and involved in this research has felt more empowering, validating and helpful than counselling would have been. I say that not just because I'm an activist and have many criticisms about counselling – I just feel that it's true.

This is, of course, a very important process for me, but I also believe it is very important research for women and part of our fight to achieve real control over our bodies.

Conclusion

I have always been quite sure that I never wanted children even as a child myself. I have never given myself the choice between having and not having a child as I have never had the slightest interest in having one. I didn't particularly think, Oh, I couldn't do all these things if I had children. It's not something I put off, or even made a choice about. (Sally)

Although still relatively unusual, it is possible for a woman to consider her future without children: increasingly, there are challenges to the belief that happiness for women comes primarily through achieving motherhood. In the West the cultural assumptions about the inevitability of motherhood are open to the criticism that a narrow view of women's future lives may deny them the opportunity to perceive and consider a range of other worthwhile and fulfilling experiences. Traditional ways of thinking about women are embedded in a legacy of cultural, historical constructions of what women are and how they should be, and 'knowing' that all women want and need children is no longer a sustainable assumption. Yet, for as long as motherhood is accepted as the most natural role for all women and the most fulfilling of achievements, any woman who openly challenges and resists what is considered as such a normal function is viewed with astonishment and may even be ignored and infantized or dismissed as dysfunctional.

The World Health Organisation has estimated that by the time that they reach age 45, 88 per cent of the world's women will have become mothers. Many of the remaining 12 per cent who experience problems conceiving will regard not having children as a loss and others, if they have the means at their disposal, will vigorously pursue the chance for motherhood. This makes it incontrovertibly the case that most women who are able to conceive a child will go on to do so although, as has been suggested in this context, having and wanting are not the same. Recent work in the field of fertility shows clear imbalances in the attitudes and behaviour towards and the treatment of the two categories of 'childfree' (women who do not want to conceive and will strenuously avoid pregnancy) and 'childless' (women who wish to yet cannot conceive or carry a baby to full term). Applications for sterilization from a childfree woman are often trivialized or dismissed, whilst the anxiety of a woman who has difficulty in becoming pregnant or carrying a baby to full term is often treated sympathetically: her desire to conceive a child is taken very seriously indeed.

Women are subject to strong messages that being a mother will be a natural, normal part of their future life, a goal to aspire to and achieve even at great physical, emotional and economic cost. In contemporary Britain the age at which a woman has her first child is rising and recent reports give clear indications that some women are choosing to delay – sometimes indefinitely – the decision to have a child at all. In this, the notion that motherhood is the destiny for all women is seriously challenged as more women are remaining childfree: from those, a small number opt for voluntary sterilization to prevent pregnancy and avoid motherhood. Such a trend gives some indication that there are women who are determined to take decisive control of their own fertility, to extend their choice beyond birth control and family planning by framing life plans based on personal decisions about their childfree future. For a small, but increasing, number of British women, motherhood is but one of a number of future destinies, as more women identify and choose to pursue radically different life goals from women of only a few decades past.

Despite the range of contraceptive choices on offer to women in the West, most have only relatively recently become available and accessible to the majority of women and there continue to be fears, particularly about oral and other chemical methods, which even the assurances of the medical profession cannot allay. When women encounter difficulties in obtaining safe and effective birth control or experience refusal or delay in abortion procedures, the consequence is that they describe feeling disempowered from controlling this vital area of their life. Given that in the past there will have been women who may have considered remaining childfree had such a choice been possible, the widening of contraceptive choice to include sterilization now allows women an expanded opportunity to consider whether or not they ever do want to have a child.

Undoubtedly, seeking an operation which is so permanent and invasive is a major decision for any woman to take. For women of any age pre-menopause, the decision not to have children demands constant monitoring of the fertility cycle and ongoing vigilance in contraceptive use. This study highlights a distinction between women who continue to use contraceptive methods until past their menopause so remaining childfree for life, and women who decided that long-term contraception had no place in their lives as it allowed an unwanted potential for motherhood. The women in this study insisted that only sterilization accurately reflected their childfree decision and permanently secured their chosen lifestyle. After sterilization, even quite young women were relieved and delighted to be able to cease taking any contraceptive precautions (although the necessity for safe sex continued) and the monthly anxieties and occasional pregnancy 'scares' disappeared.

What has emerged very clearly from this study is that at the heart of all applications for elective sterilization (from childfree women, women with children and also from men) is an overriding dissatisfaction with currently available contraception. Despite very considerable usage of contraceptive methods, which offer less of a choice than is generally believed, many women remain desperately worried about unwanted pregnancy. Depending on the method used, sterilization has a failure rate of one to three in a thousand compared with just under one in a hundred for the Pill: this means that sterilization is almost ten times more effective than oral contraception. The women in this study who had undergone sterilization commenced their sexual lives wanting safe and effective contraception and freedom from the fear of unplanned and unwanted pregnancies. Having tried other methods, all of which were or became unsuitable in some way, they decided that only sterilization was able to provide security and peace of mind. In their terms, as women determined to remain childfree, they considered that any contraceptive which offered only 99 per cent protection was not good enough.

For women even to begin to consider remaining childfree a number of significant social factors should ideally exist and be available as options even if they are contested and challenged. In order to make a personal choice to remain childfree and then to be able to act upon that decision through elective sterilization, it is likely that the following five factors would need to be in place within any culture and society. They already feature in structurally complex Western lifestyles, and also can be identified and observed in countries and societies which are capital intense, highly industrialized and technologically sophisticated.

1. Women must have the unquestioned right to define their sexual identity and the rights and opportunities to remain independent of a man and unmarried;
2. they must have opportunities for economic independence, realizable through educational success, and access to paid work;
3. they must have the right and opportunity to consider remaining childfree and to have opportunities for a complete and final say over all aspects of their reproductive lives;
4. they must have access to safe and effective contraception and, if unplanned pregnancies occur, must have the right and opportunity to opt for early and safe abortion; and
5. they must have access to contraception and, if they choose to cease using contraceptive methods, must have the right and opportunity to opt for sterilization regardless of whether they have had children.

By telling their stories and describing their experiences, the childfree sterilized women in this study provided the material and detail for the five factors, although these are not intended to be definitive or final. Rather they may be useful as guidelines for identifying the necessary social conditions and cultural context within which women may more easily make choices and reach decisions which they feel are best for them as individuals and which many of them also considered to be in the interests of society.

Many of the sterilized childfree women in this book expressed feelings of isolation and of being 'out of step' with other women, they even felt they were not 'real' women. Most commented, either in diaries or during interviews, at feeling relief on discovering that there were other women who felt as they had, and who had been sterilized. Other studies show women who, as a result of their lifestyle, realized that they preferred living without children: continuing to live without children developed as a consequence of the way that they chose to live their lives. In this important regard, a crucial difference emerged between childfree women who continue to depend upon contraception and the voices and experiences of the majority of this study's childfree, electively sterilized women, who emphasized that they had 'always known' that they did not want children and had placed being childfree at the forefront of planning how their lives would be lived.

In social contexts in which motherhood is perceived as being the only natural outcome of an instinctual desire, women who determine not to have children are perceived as abnormal and unnatural. Childfree women seem to be capable of exploring and affirming their decision without the support of an independent outsider, such as a counsellor, an attribute that becomes increasingly important. This is because, as they reach the decision to cease using method contraception and consider sterilization, they cannot fail to become aware of the disapproval and opposition which they face and must overcome before being able to progress and act on their decision. It would seem that doctors and consultants make a negative assessment of the childfree status of a woman who makes the approach, based on an unresearched and untested assumption that her childfree choice is one which will inevitably change as she gets older, leading to her regretting the decision and returning for reversal of the procedure.

Even within the field of medical research itself there is sufficient evidence to indicate that childfree women are much less likely to regret their decision or to request reversal and that it is more likely that they have reached their decision early in life and not wavered in their resolve. In this regard, they are different from some other women who perhaps do not make a conscious decision against motherhood, but who postpone having a child until they find – regretfully or with relief – that they have simply run out of biological time. However, it is acknowledged that the small number of women in this study means that they may be seen as an unrepresentative and self-selected sample and that there are, indeed, childfree women who opted for sterilization and who – like Heather – now deeply regret the decision.

From the outset of any request for sterilization from a childfree woman, the GPs and the doctors and specialists who deal with fertility insist that she spend time considering how serious and irreversible is the decision she has reached. The caution expressed by doctors is understandable but studies, including this one, do show that some women are aware from early on in their lives that they have no wish to have a child.

Therefore, demands that they 'go away and think about it' suggest that doctors may believe there to be only a short time between the woman deciding to be sterilized and her making an application. The timescale between avoiding pregnancy and motherhood and considering being sterilized supported the assertion by childfree women that they had already made their decision to remain childfree a number of years prior to the decision to be sterilized. Also, they make a decision which is different from women who also do not intend having children but continue to use and depend on monthly contraception as, before considering sterilization, they also knew that they did not want children, needed to continue protecting against unwanted pregnancy, but wanted to stop using contraceptive methods. Further, women who are determined to remain childfree frequently express high levels of concern and anxiety about the unsatisfactory and unsafe methods of contraception used and this dissatisfaction is a major factor in deciding to opt for sterilization.

Women who are clear that they do not want to have children and say so openly attract disapproval and censure and may be seen as abnormal, or considered to be not 'real' women. They often face disapproval and refusal from doctors and consultants, encountering barriers and difficulties with the medical profession as soon as they seek information about sterilization and feel that, despite their usually mature age, they are not considered to be capable of making a decision about sterilization as a method of controlling their own fertility.

Childfree women and women who are mothers have different motivations for deciding on sterilization, although they appear to be taking the same course of action for an identical outcome. None of the women wants to become pregnant and it is likely that there are similar feelings of relief between the two groups at being able to give up monthly birth control precautions. The difference is, however, that mothers want no more children but childfree women want no children at all. This difference is usually not acknowledged and is often considered as unimportant and ignored or dismissed by GPs and consultants. In this way it appears that the return rate for reversals and the reasons given by sterilized women who are mothers – mainly so that they can try to have more children – is used as part of the medical excuses for decisions not to sterilize women who state their determination to remain childfree, although childfree women who say that they have 'always known' that they do not want children are less likely to apply for reversal than sterilized women who have had children.

Despite medical and social disapproval, childfree women believe that they have a right to take decisions about their own bodies, yet attempting to act upon their determination is fraught with hazards and obstacles even for determined, highly articulate women, who face a slow-to-change resistance from the medical world. Stripped of the moral disapproval it currently attracts, sterilization becomes only one of the many available methods of contraception. Elective sterilization offers the best chance of permanently preventing pregnancy and unwanted entry into the state of motherhood and is the method which currently offers the highest degree of security and peace of mind to determinedly childfree women.

For some women to be able to choose and define personal life goals and roles (in this instance, long-term contraception and remaining childfree) and implementing decisions which arise from such choices (in this instance, undergoing sterilization) is one consequence of the result of rapid advances made in the reproductive technologies especially over the past 40 years. The benefits of this are incalculable and women have been released from the annual round of exhausting and debilitating unplanned pregnancies and childbearing followed by years in which they concentrate on child-rearing. Increasingly, opportunities appear to be available for relationships which are more balanced and egalitarian than those presented within the traditional model of family life and fuller, richer lives which could allow women more positive experiences of mothering so that, rather than having to make all or nothing decisions between career or family, it is possible to have children and to maintain other interests and activities. Nevertheless, some women assert that choosing motherhood was never an option for them, that their decision not to have children was a positive one and their commitment to a childfree lifestyle is ongoing and not regretted.

The women in this study knew from an early age that they did not want to become mothers and did not intend to spend their fertile lives fearful of pregnancy and preventing conception by barrier and chemical methods. The decision to be sterilized was a consequence and, for them, the logical outcome of being childfree. They did not choose to be sterilized in order not to have a child as that choice had been made earlier in their lives; thus, sterilization was the final choice of contraception for the 23 women in this study. They argued for, and achieved, their personal right to make essential decisions about their own fertility and reproductive capacity by avoiding motherhood and choosing sterilization. Such resistance may contribute to demystifying and weakening the powerful ideologies of what it is to be 'woman' and 'mother' as, in their individually unique ways, they opposed traditions which they felt to be oppressive and challenged what seemed to them to be unquestioned ideologies. In doing so and electing for sterilization in order to remain childfree, these women made clear that they were prepared to act on their own decisions, for their own reasons and in their own interests.

Appendix: Selected Responses from the Questionnaire and Transcribed Interviews

Sexuality: contraception, pregnancies, sterilization

In response to the question asking the respondents to describe their sexual identity, twelve of the 23 women identified themselves as 'heterosexual'. A further seven women wrote that they were heterosexual but went on to use a qualifying phrases such as 'mainly' or 'mostly', or commented 'haven't tried anything else'. Three women said that they had had sexual experiences, or had had a relationship with other women at some time in their lives, and one woman who identified as lesbian said that she had lived a heterosexual lifestyle until her mid-thirties.

All of the women had used some form of contraception during their lives and most had continued with the method they were using up to and immediately preceding the sterilization operation. Of the 23 sterilized women, 22 had used the Pill or mini pill and one could not use the Pill. As alternatives to the Pill and usually during periods of celibacy (or what they described as 'breaks' because of unease at continued pill use) women also said that they made use of: diaphragm (cap) and contraceptive jelly (2); condoms (5); IUD, various types (5); 'withdrawal' and unprotected sex (3); non-penetrative sex (1).

Nine women mentioned incidences of pregnancy: one ectopic pregnancy; two miscarriages of unplanned pregnancies; four women had had one abortion each; one woman had had four abortions which she blamed on contraceptive failure; one baby had been adopted shortly after its birth. Ten women mentioned 'one', 'some', 'several' or 'frequent' scares, including one who resorted to taking the morning-after pill. Four women mentioned that they would have had an abortion if the pregnancy scare had been real.

Fourteen women were sterilized in NHS hospitals and nine women in private hospitals. Help and advice by Marie Stopes Clinics was mentioned by four women. The sterilization methods used were (using the women's own descriptions): tubes tied (2); tubal ligation (5); clips (11); cauterization (3); coagulation (1); does not know (1).

The reasons for opting to be sterilized were integral to every woman's interview and diary. Some answered the question directly and the following extracts are from the responses of the fourteen women who most clearly identified their reasons for considering giving up contraceptive methods and applying for sterilization. The two outstanding reasons given are (i) fear of pregnancy or a 'scare' and/or (ii) disliking, mistrusting or finding other contraceptive methods irrelevant because they had 'always known' that they did not want children. The following comments from fourteen women are taken from the tape recordings of interviews or taken from the diaries.

> The decision to ask for sterilization was made finally when it was necessary for me to have a break after such a long time on the Pill. The contraceptive options were cap, coil, or sheath and spermicide. We tried the latter for a month before I went back on the Pill and asked for sterilization. (Geraldine)

> I was three weeks late with my period and facing abortion – a position I never wanted to be in in the first place. So when I tested negative, much to my relief, I TOLD my GP I wanted to be sterilized. (Linda L.)

> I'd decided not to have a child so it seemed the obvious thing to do – I didn't want to be on the Pill any longer than I needed to be – although I never had unpleasant side effects it just didn't seem a good idea to be eating hormones indefinitely! (Judith)

> I was unable to take the oral contraceptive pill and wanted a reliable contraceptive method. (Gillian)

> Sterilization is the only answer to the unsatisfactory contraceptive methods I had been using. (Jude)

> I wanted to be sterilized because I didn't want to keep taking

chemicals to control my fertility when I didn't need it at all. (Sandy)

After going through all the 'failure' rate statistics I made it clear to the consultant that I was sure that sterilization was what I wanted. (Vicky)

From the age of 18 up to about 28 I had taken the contraceptive pill but had become disturbed by the ever-increasing reports of associated health risks. (Heather)

My reason was to be certain of not conceiving as I was unhappy with the Pill and IUD. My decision to be sterilized didn't seem major then or now, just a logical and simple form of contraception. (Jill)

I lived in fear of my body ambushing me . . . It's the permanence and peace of mind of sterilization that I want to attain and reading around the subject has made me more confident that this is what I want. (Gemma: from a letter to a consultant)

There was a real fear of pregnancy and I experienced problems with medication because of the Pill. (Ginny)

It was essential to ensure no conflict about potential motherhood with future partners. (Liz)

I found it quite easy to make the decision to be sterilized and do not recall any problems about it. My husband was supportive – we did not want any children and it seemed the logical thing to do. (Linda R.)

I had been asking about sterilization since I became sexually active at 17 and went to the family planning service. I was told I was too young and would change my mind when I was older. I was sterilized because I never want children and therefore didn't see the point in using contraceptives for the rest of my fertile life – particularly as nothing is 100 per cent. (Helen)

'I'd always known that I didn't want children . . .'

Fifteen women responded at length in diaries and during interviews to the question asking when each had first known or acknowledged that she did not want to have children: the other women made more oblique references, often using the phrase 'I just always knew'. Several of the diarists also spoke with feeling about their childhood experiences, their relationships with their mothers or contributed observations of what they felt to be the drudgery of their mother's lives, revealing that they had had or were having 'difficulties' of some kind in their relationships with their mothers. Whilst I do not intend to imply that the mothers were 'bad', or in any way abusive or destructive (other than what I was told in the quotations included below), it is tempting to speculate (as the question was not asked at interview) that so-called 'normal' mothering in itself has elements which may be experienced as alienating and deeply distressing to children. It could be that these women were particularly sensitive to aspects of their mother's 'mothering' in ways which reinforced, not just the message to be mother, but that to be 'mother' was not a choice that they wished to make. Adrienne Rich uses 'matrophobia' which may, in part, describe this, as it is taken to mean not to fear being a mother, and not to fear one's own mother, but a fear of becoming one's own mother (Rich, 1976).

Nancy Chodorow's 'object relations' theory is also of interest, as she concentrated on the ways in which girls focus on their mothers in order to learn how to become women and mothers. She also acknowledged that there is a tension within the processes through which mothering is reproduced and argued that in order to construct a theory of motherhood it was necessary to recognize that the 'perfect mother' is a myth (in Gordon, 1990).

> As far as I can remember I've always known I didn't want children and this was confirmed after a late period scare. I have never had any kind of maternal urge. I have discussed and explored this and listened to friends who have, or who greatly want – and have failed – to have children. I simply don't share the feelings. (Jill)

> I was always aware that I didn't want children. There may have been a point when I was first married when I might have caved in and had one to conform, but I could see how much having children drained my mother as a person, so I've always known I didn't want kids – this feeling just got stronger the older I got and has been reinforced by my life experiences. (Linda L.)

> I have never wanted children and made a formal decision at 14

that I wouldn't have any. I can't recall any bigger factors, but babies have never had any appeal. (Gillian)

I've always known that children were not for me. I can't remember anything other than knowing that. (Anne D.)

I just always knew from my teenage years that I did not want children. (Liz)

I didn't want children and couldn't imagine children in my life. (Anne T.)

I can't remember when I first identified that I didn't want a child. I think I've always known and it is linked with the question of my sexual identity. When I was younger my landlady would pour out her heart about a son who abandoned her as soon as he married. At 18, I thought, 'I'm never having children . . .' (Pauline)

I have always, always known that I didn't want to have children. Probably since the age of fourteen or fifteen years I have had an awareness and growing feminist conviction of women's issues. I have never ever felt differently or had a so-called 'broody' phase. I want always to be childfree. (Jude)

I planned a career in the Church. As a teenager I wanted to be a Deaconess. At that time they weren't allowed to marry so I never considered having children. (Jean)

I was just always generally aware and the main reason I didn't have children was that I was just too busy – I had almost an addiction to sport, and really was not maternal at all. (Lesley)

I have never wanted children. The following explanation took me over thirty years to work out, but my mother taught me to hate children by the way she treated me. I coped with it as a child by rationalizing that it wasn't me she hated, she only treated me that way because I was a child, and that if I could only grow up and be an adult then it would all be OK. (Helen)

There was a very strong reason for not wanting children and part of it was to do with the intrusive nature of my mother into my life. I wasn't the 'right' daughter. Early on I was aware that when you have a child you are inviting and introducing a stranger into your life. (Vicky)

During my teens, I just felt that I did not want to be trapped. That was how I saw my own mother, putting her children first for a good part of her useful life. (Ginny)

I have always known I didn't want children. With hindsight I feel that it is to do with the way that I saw my father controlling mother. (Geraldine)

I do not have any strong maternal feelings . . . I fear that, because I was rejected as a baby, there is every likelihood that I would subject a child to this rejection. (Gemma: from a letter to a consultant)

Relief and regret

Nineteen women responded to the final question, identifying their current feelings as childfree women after being sterilized. The short sentence 'I have never had a single regret' was used by many and so not all are included, and the main text of the book may contain more of the quotation than is given here.

I had no doubts at all and don't regret not having children. (Lesley)

After the op. I was REALLY happy, so relieved to not have to take precautions, not to have chemicals in my body. I remain delighted with and totally committed to my decision. (Sandy)

It was agreed that I could have the sterilization as well as the abortion. That was eleven years ago and I have never regretted either the decision or the operation. (Christine)

I never thought of giving up, or changing my mind, and I have never had any regrets. (Jean)

I'm my own woman and I never live with regret, I'm good at not regretting decisions. My life would have been terribly different if I'd had children, especially after my marriage broke up. Because I like children I think that I have the best of both worlds, as I can form relationships with those kids that I like. (Sally)

I have no regrets, in fact I feel totally relieved and liberated. It has been a wonderful thing for me and it has been so nice to come off the Pill and not have the fear of pregnancy hanging over me. (Jude)

I have never regretted the decision, it is a great relief, but I wonder what motherhood might have been like. (Pauline)

I am sure that if I hadn't been sterilized (my present husband and I) would have seriously considered having a child – mostly it was a relief that we didn't need to get into heavy discussions about children as the decision was made and that was that! But I did get occasional pangs of wistfulness [because of the negative experience of pregnancy as a teenager]. (Judith)

Counselling experiences

The following are statements given by the twenty women who responded to the question asking for experiences of counselling for or about sterilization, using their own interpretation of the term.

I didn't consult my GP or ask for referral. He was less than helpful with advice about alternative contraception after advising me to stop taking the Pill. I was not counselled as such. When I was referred, I saw a man who asked me whether I was pregnant and told me that a D&C would be necessary in addition to the sterilization. I discussed my reasons – and that was that! I accepted that I would not have children in this lifetime. Having a belief in reincarnation helps, it puts it all in perspective. (Linda R.)

Counselling was not offered before or after and if it had been I doubt I would have accepted it. I believe I would have viewed it as a method designed to stop me getting the sterilization. (Geraldine)

I did not seek counselling in any form as I was comfortable with the decision. (Liz)

I got it through the NHS, which I didn't expect to be so easy, but it only took a few months from discussing it with the GP to getting a hospital date. If I hadn't been sure, it wouldn't have been very long to think about things, but I probably made it clear to the GP that I had thought about it and was sure! I didn't get any 'professional' advice. The GP gave me leaflets to read and come back in

2 weeks if I was still sure. At the time of the operation I can remember a 'this-is-what-we-do' kind of conversation. I am a quiet but assertive person and probably gave out messages that I had thought it through and didn't want further discussion. (Judith)

I never 'consulted' anybody except my GP to achieve sterilization but I've discussed the idea with friends and family and, of course, my partner who wanted to reassure and be reassured it wasn't a decision for his benefit only and that I was 100 per cent sure and happy about it. (Linda L.)

I discussed my decision with my mother and with my Church. I never visited a counsellor. (Ginny)

I did discuss my decision with my mother who, because of my age, was very supportive. (Pauline)

Marie Stopes provided 'professional' counselling and I felt that they asked the right questions and provided appropriate information. The counselling was mostly questions which you ought to be able to answer, 'are you sure . . .' etc. but also involved a full description of the methods. It was quite gentle really. I don't think I've had a burning need to explore why I don't want children, it's been more that other people seem to react to it. In my own counselling I thought well, perhaps there is something that I should explore, but I didn't find out anything that I didn't know, although it was interesting enough. (Jill)

I was able to get the essential and necessary information very easily and the process, on the whole, was smooth and untroubled apart from the after-effects of the ovarian cyst operation which were not really connected with the sterilization. My discussion with a female friend was very positive. (Anne T.)

My family were and still are very much of the opinion that one makes one's bed, so my decision was not opposed or much discussed. I attended the consultation alone as my husband's presence didn't seem wanted or necessary. I think, at the time, I would not have welcomed discussion and certainly did not seek 'advice' on the issue. My family and friends just accepted that, if I had made up my mind, there wasn't much point in trying to persuade me otherwise. (Heather)

My husband had been married before in a childfree marriage. The decision for me to be sterilized was our decision and was not discussed with anyone else. (Gillian)

I had 5 minutes 'counselling' prior to the operation. (Helen)

I do think that exploring my decision to be childfree in my mid-twenties might have been useful, which is the start of the time when people ask why you haven't got children, or when are you going to have them. I could then, perhaps, have identified and explored my own internalized 'stuff' and, in a more clear way, been able to stand by what I had always wanted and felt. I didn't have counselling mainly because I was so clear – I'd have wanted a feminist debate around how people responded. I am a counsellor so I have had counselling, but never brought this as an 'issue'. In retrospect I WOULD have liked counselling AFTER sterilization was agreed – people's responses were so awful and I needed help to deal with that, not the decision. I wanted to be round other women who had been sterilized so we could compare notes about how bad people were. I needed to explore and direct my anger and that's why taking part in this [research] has been so important to me. It's given me an opportunity to talk about the whole process in a feminist way with another feminist. For me, it's been the place for that support and where to channel that anger, much more than counselling would be. (Jude)

I think it is very important to seek the support of friends or family whilst still retaining privacy and control over how many, or how much, people know. For the most part I told only those from whom I was confident of support and I was not disappointed or betrayed. At the hospital the female consultant delivered a 'pep talk' then gave me a quick internal examination. (Gemma)

I didn't visit a counsellor but don't feel it would have helped. I did discuss my decision with my husband, friends and my mother, and took 'professional' advice on methods from the local family planning clinic. My mother was supportive and my friends all said they couldn't imagine me with kids anyway! The 'advice' came from the consultant, and friends who said 'You lucky bugger!' – but no counselling about whether to, or discussing what was already my decision. (Sandy)

Apart from 'are you sure' type of questions there was nothing at all though if they'd said 'you've got to have counselling' I'd have gone. I am a counsellor as are most of my friends so there would have been support. It all seemed very straightforward so I don't think I would have found it useful. (Jean)

I did have a discussion with the gynaecologist and there was a bit of repartee . . . but nothing that could be counted as counselling about being childfree. (Vicky)

I felt no need to talk to anyone else about it as I wasn't looking for anyone to help me come to a decision or to confirm my decision for me. (Sally)

I've never really needed counselling because my mind has always been made up. (Christine)

Because of her regrets after the sterilization and her application for reversal, Heather found that she was subject to the type of counselling which she described as being 'very disapproving':

The mythical 'counselling' was alluded to many times, such as, 'after all the counselling you had before the operation which was supposed to ensure that this wouldn't happen' and so on. In the end I just had to say I didn't GET any! I wasn't blaming anyone else for making the wrong decision. I accept fully that it was all down to me, but I did begin to resent the implication that, despite all the NHS had put in on my behalf, I wanted on a whim to cause them some more trouble! I was treated to a lurid description of the complexity of the operation (something I wasn't given about the actual sterilization) complete with dire warnings. If his directive is to dissuade all prospective candidates for reversal, he should be commended for his efforts! (Heather)

Glossary

Some of the following may be familiar, especially acronyms and medical terminology. Family Planning Association literature was helpful for brief and concise information. Other words in the list have lengthy comments, especially where descriptions of concepts seems necessary, or where I seek to explain my choice and use of particular terms.

BON British Organisation for Non-parents.* An Edinburgh-based group which reports that it has a high turnover group of around 150 members at any time. It developed out of ISSUE (c.f.) which did not sufficiently represent the needs of the childfree, its original title attracting those who were involuntarily without children. Membership tends to be short-lived. The chairman, Root Cartwright, says, '[the couples] get involved when it's a hot issue for them, in the throes of the decision-making process, or being given a hard time by families' (in Jane Bartlett, *Will You Be Mother?*, 1994).

BPAS British Pregnancy Advisory Service. A national non-profit-making charity, founded in 1967 after the passing of the Abortion Act, in order to meet the needs of women seeking help and advice about abortion. Currently there are seven clinics which also provide counselling and fertility-related medical treatment and may work with the NHS to provide a free service.

childfree The term most used by women and preferred by myself, rather than childless. Both, of course, place 'child' first, appearing to denote an absence or lack of something rather than a positive choice. I comment on this uncomfortable position in the book.

contraceptive methods The Family Planning Association defines methods currently in use worldwide as: combined and progesterone-only oral contraceptive pill (with ongoing trials for a male pill); male and female condoms; diaphragm; cap; injectables; implants (e.g. Norplant); natural family planning (including the latest, Persona, which in 1997–98 is showing a very high 'failure' rate); intrauterine devices (e.g. coil, or Copper 7); intrauterine system (IUD plus slow hormone release); female sterilization; and male vasectomy.

D&C   Dilation and curettage: a medical procedure whereby the cervix is dilated and the womb 'scraped'. Sometimes used prior to the sterilization operation to ensure that there is no implanted embryo.

diarists   A term I use to describe the 23 childfree sterilized women in the study. Jane was interviewed and did not write her story.

ectopic pregnancy   A dangerous condition, and life-threatening if not quickly dealt with, whereby a fertilized egg begins to develop within a fallopian tube, leading to intense pain and eventual rupture and possibly causing permanent damage. Sperm are considerably smaller than the ovum and so are able to swim through the narrow passage of the fallopian tube and fertilize a ripe ovum but the fertilized ovum cannot then pass along the tube into the uterus and implant. As sterilization effectively blocks the passage of any fertilized egg travelling to the womb, there is a higher incidence of ectopic pregnancies in sterilized women.

eugenics   'The study of methods of improving the quality of the human race especially by selective breeding' (Collins *English Dictionary*).

(UN)FPA   (United Nations) Family Planning Association.

feminist research   'The aim of feminist research is to create theories grounded in the actual experiences and language of women by. investigating women's lives and experience in their own terms . . . In addition, feminist research courts subjective involvement in its bid to gain new theoretical understanding' (Humm, 1989).

fertility   Feminist theories posit that this is not just the ability of women to produce children but is a major component of sexual power relations between women and men and may be studied from historical, political and psychological perspectives. Robyn Rowland (1992) warns that coerced motherhood is the result of women having no right not to reproduce. Rosalind Petchesky (international coordinator, International Reproductive Rights Research Action Group) says that women desire to know and be in control of their own bodies and this leads on to a consideration of reproductive rights which includes not only the right to become a mother (a 'rights' issue which is contested) but also the rights to have access to a full range of contraceptive and birth control methods, including abortion and, this study will assert, the right to elect for sterilization.

Filshie clip Rapidly becoming the favoured clip for female sterilization. Developed by and named after Nottinghamshire gynaecologist Dr Marcus Filshie.

hysterectomy The only irreversible and permanent method of sterilization. May involve total removal of uterus, ovaries and fallopian tubes, or be partial, where the ovaries (if healthy) remain in order to prevent the onset of early menopause. Although suitable for specific medical conditions, it is nowadays considered to be a drastic method of sterilization in otherwise healthy women, although it retains its medical 'popularity' when women complain about heavy periods or where the womb has fibroids. (A book which challenges the overuse of this medical procedure is *No More Hysterectomies* by Dr Vicki Hufnagel, 1990.)

infantizing I made use of a model of 'infantilization' (Karen A. Lyman (1996) 'Infantilization: the medical model of care', in *Perspectives in Medical Sociology*, ed. Phil Brown, pp. 299–309). It has a high correlation with the reception afforded to the requests of childfree women when they were making initial inquiries and applications for sterilization, and is significant in that it accords with the use of the description 'infantized' as used in a number of the diaries and at interview with the participants. The model uses six methods of control over the patients: (i) directives, (ii) deception, (iii) careful coercion (including distraction and behaviour modification), (iv) pharmacological restraints, (v) segregation, (vi) environmental control. Not every method was applicable in the form originally envisaged, but the concept of control of consultants over patients was useful to bear in mind in the scrutiny and critical assessment of replies to the question.

IPPF International Planned Parenthood Federation.

ISSUE The national fertility association. Its primary aim is to provide information and support for the one in six couples who have trouble conceiving.

laparoscopy The most common method of sterilization and the most quoted method by the women in this study. The fallopian tubes are reached by one or two tiny cuts (below navel and in 'bikini-line') and a thin, telescope-like surgical instrument with magnifying lenses (the laparoscope) is inserted. The fallopian tubes are sealed or blocked, sometimes with rings or clips, or they may be cut and tied, or sealed by coagulation or cauterization (women sometimes use the terms 'tubes tied' or 'tubes burnt'). (I found of interest the short history of sterilization methods, described in Clive Wood's (1974) *Vasectomy and Sterilization: A Guide for Men and Women*, Chapter 3; also IPPF, *Family Planning Handbook for Doctors*, Chapter 11).

ligation The fallopian tubes are reached and blocked by tying (ligation) and then removing a small piece of tube (excision).

Marie Stopes International A registered charity working in 25 countries with the objective of providing 'high quality, sustainable services at a price which is affordable to all' (information leaflet, 1996). The first family planning clinic was opened by Marie Stopes in 1921, despite criticism and outrage by the conservative medical and religious establishment in response to her outspoken advocacy of contraception.

nulliparous woman A woman who has not borne a child.

reversal The surgical attempt to repair the effects of sterilization. This may involve removal of the clips or rings on the fallopian tubes or attempts to reopen the tubes in order to allow a fertilized egg to travel to the womb. Whilst all of the services offering sterilization emphasize that it should be considered to be irreversible, BPAS includes the cost of reversal on their price list for both female sterilization (£1,575) and male vasectomy (£1,015).

second-wave feminism 'A term coined by Marsha Wienman Lear to refer to the formation of women's liberation groups in America, Britain and Germany in the late 1960s. The term "second wave" implies that "first wave" feminism ended in the 1920s' (Humm, 1989).

sterilization Used usually to describe the variety of ways in which a woman may be operated upon in order to prevent pregnancy.

Works by preventing any fertilized ovum travelling from the fallopian tubes and implanting in the womb. (My discussions with consultant gynaecologists and other medical professionals indicated that the method used was likely to be the personal preference of each individual surgeon.)

TOP Termination of pregnancy: abortion.

---

* The organization BON provides a starting point for those who may be questioning whether or not they want to become parents, especially if they feel themselves to be under pressure from relatives and friends. The range of information material provides the type of questions that few people ever hear asked openly, much less discussed when what is usually heard emphasizes the natural state of parenthood. Three useful leaflets from the organization are *You Do Have a Choice!*, *Am I Parent Material?* and *No Regrets*. These are not anti-child but contain questions encouraging all people to think deeply and responsibly about bringing new life into the world, and the consequent new responsibilities towards child, partner and society itself.

Bibliography

Acker, Sandra (1994) *Gendered Education*. Buckingham: Open University Press.

Allen, Isobel (1981) *Family Planning, Sterilisation and Abortion Services*. London: Policy Studies Institute.

Allen, Isobel (1985) *Counselling Services For Sterilisation, Vasectomy, and Termination of Pregnancy*. London: Policy Studies Institute.

Allen, Jeffner (1983) 'Motherhood: the annihilation of women', in Joyce Trebilcot (ed.), *Mothering: Essays in Feminist Theory*. Washington, Maryland: Rowland & Littlefield.

Badinter, Elisabeth (1981) *The Myth of Motherhood: An Historical View of the Maternal Instinct*. London: Souvenir Press.

Bandura, A. (1977) *Social Learning Theory*. Englewood Cliffs, NJ: Prentice Hall.

Barrett, Jane *et al.* (eds) (1985) *Vukani Makhosikazi: South African Women Speak*. Springs, SA: Catholic Institute for International Relations (CIIR).

Barrett, Michele (1980) *Women's Oppression Today*. London: Verso.

Bart, Pauline (1979) 'Review of Chodorow's *The Reproduction of Mothering*', in Joyce Trebilcot (ed) *Mothering: Essays in Feminist Theory*. Washington, Maryland: Rowland & Littlefield.

Bartlett, Jane (1994) *Will You Be Mother?: Women Who Choose To Say No*. London: Virago.

Baum, F. and Cope, D. (1980) 'Some characteristics of intentionally childless wives in Britain', *Biosocial Science*, 12, 287–99.

Beechey, Veronica (1979) 'On patriarchy', *Feminist Review*, 3.

Belotti, Elena Gianni (1975) *Little Girls*. London: Writers' and Readers' Publishing Cooperative.

Bem, Sandra (1974) 'The measurement of psychological androgyny', *Journal of Consulting and Clinical Psychology*, 42, 155–62.

Bepko, Claudia and Krestan, Jo-Ann (1990) *Too Good for Her Own Good: Searching for Self and Intimacy in Important Relationships*. New York: HarperPerennial.

Bernard, Jessie (1974) *The Future of Motherhood*. New York: The Dial Press.

Besant, Annie (n.d.) *The Law of Population: its Consequences, and its Bearing Upon Human Conduct and Morals*. London: Freethought Publishing Company.

Birmingham Evening Mail (1996) 'Failed op. mum to sue over baby', 28 Dec. 1996.

Birmingham Evening Mail, (1997) 'Price of protection', 23 Jan. 1997.

Bleir, Ruth (1984) *Science and Gender: A Critique of Biology and its Theories of Women*. Oxford: Pergamon.

Boston Women's Health Book Collective (1971) *Our Bodies Ourselves: A Health Book by and for Women*. Harmondsworth: Penguin Books.

Bowlby, John (1965) *Child Care and the Growth of Love*. Harmondsworth: Penguin Books.

Bowles, G. and Duelli Klein, R. (eds) (1983) *Theories of Women's Studies*. London: Routledge and Kegan Paul.

Boyle, M. (1992) 'The abortion debate', in Paula Nicolson and Jane Ussher (eds), *The Psychology of Women's Health and Health Care*. London: Macmillan.

Brierley, John (1987) *'Give Me a Child until He is Seven . . .': Brain Studies and Early Childhood Education*. East Sussex: The Falmer Press.

British Association for Counselling (BAC) (1995) 'Training in counselling' (information sheets, October). Rugby: BAC.

Brooks, Ann (1997) *Postfeminisms: Feminism, Cultural Theory and Cultural Forms*. New York and London: Routledge.

Brown, Phil (ed.) (1996) (2nd edn) *Perspectives in Medical Sociology*. Illinois: Waveland Press.

Brownmiller, Susan (1975) *Against Our Will: Men, Women, and Rape*. New York: Simon and Schuster.

Bryson, Valerie (1992) *Feminist Political Theory: An Introduction*. London: Macmillan.

Burgess, R. G. (1995) (4th edn.) *In the Field: An Introduction to Field Research*. London: Routledge.

Burgwyn, Diana (1981) *Marriage Without Children*. New York: Harper and Row.

Burman, Erica (ed.) (1990) *Feminists and Psychological Practice*. London: Sage.

Butler, Judith (1990) *Gender Trouble: Feminism and the Subversion of Identity*. New York and London: Routledge.

Caldwell, Jack (1982) *Theory of Fertility Decline*. London: Academic Press.

Campbell, Annily C. (1998) ' "From the wilder shores of the feminist movement": Childfree sterilized women challenging the "Motherhood Continuum" '. Paper presented at Women's Studies Network Conference, University of Hull.

Campbell, Elaine (1985) *The Childless Marriage: An Exploratory Study of Couples who do not Want Children*. London: Tavistock.

Cartwright, Ann (1976) *How Many Children?* London: Routledge and Kegan Paul.

Central Statistical Office (1993) *Social Trends*. London: HMSO.

Central Statistical Office (1995) *Social Trends*. London: HMSO.

Central Statistical Office (1996) *Social Trends*. London: HMSO.

Chandler, Joan (1991) *Women Without Husbands: An Exploration of the Margins of Marriage*. London: Macmillan.

Chaplin, Jocelyn (1992) *Feminist Counselling in Action*. London: Sage Publications.

Charles, Nickie (1993) *Gender Divisions and Social Change*. London: Harvester Wheatsheaf.

Chester, G. and Neilson, S. (eds) (1987) *In Other Words: Writing as a Feminist*. London: Hutchinson.

Chodorow, Nancy (1978) *The Reproduction of Mothering: Psychoanalysis and the Sociology of Gender*. Berkeley: University of California Press.

Cipola, Carlo (1962) *The Economic History of World Population*. Harmondsworth: Perguin Books.

Cockerham, William C. (1995) (6th edn.) *Medical Sociology*. New Jersey: Prentice Hall.

Cohen, L. and Manion, L. (1994) *Research Methods in Education*. London: Routledge.

Colony, Nikki (1989) 'The politics of birth control in a reproductive rights context', in Christine Overall (ed.) *The Future of Human Reproduction*. Toronto: Women's Press.

Condy, Ann (1995) 'Choosing not to have children', *Family Policy Bulletin* (April), London: Family Policy Studies Centre.

Corea, Gena (1985) *The Mother Machine: From Artificial Insemination to Artificial Wombs*. London: Women's Press.

Crowley, Helen and Himmelweit, Susan (eds) (1992) *Knowing Women: Feminism and Knowledge*. Cambridge: Policy Press; and Milton Keynes: Open University.

Cunningham-Burley, Sarah and McKeganey, Neil P. (eds) (1990) *Readings in Medical Sociology*. London: Routledge.

Dally, Ann (1982) *Inventing Motherhood: The Consequences of an Ideal*. London: Burnett Books.

Daly, Mary (1978) *Gyn/Ecology: The Metaethics of Radical Feminism*. Boston, MA: Beacon Press.

Davenport, G. C. (1988) *An Introduction to Child Development*. London: Unwin Hyman.

Davies, Miranda (ed.) (1987) *Third World – Second Sex* (Vol. 2). London: Zed Books.

Davies, Vanessa (1991) *Abortion and Afterwards*. Avon: Ashgrove Press.

Dawkins, Richard (1989) (2nd edn.) *The Selfish Gene*. Oxford: Oxford University Press.

de Beauvoir, Simone (1953) *The Second Sex*. Hermondsworth: Penguin Books.

de Lauretis, Teresa (ed.) (1986) *Feminist Studies/Critical Studies*. London: Macmillan.

Department of Health and Social Security (1984) *Report of the Committee of Inquiry into Human Fertilisation and Embryology* (Baroness Mary Warnock). London: HMSO.

Deutsch, Helene (1944) *The Psychology of Women: Vol. 1, Girlhood*. USA: Bantam Books.

Deutsch, Helene (1944) *The Psychology of Women: Vol. 2, Motherhood*. USA: Bantam Books.

Dowrick, Stephanie and Grundberg, Sybil (eds) (1980) *Why Children?*. London: Women's Press.

Ehrenreich, Barbara and English, Deirdre (1979) *For Her Own Good: 150 Years of the Experts' Advice to Women*. London: Pluto Press.

Ehrlich, Paul R. (1971) *The Population Bomb*. London: Ballantine/Friends of the Earth.

Eichler, Margrit (1988) *Nonsexist Research Methods: A Practical Guide*. London: Allen and Unwin.

Eversley, D. and Kollmann, W. (eds) (1982) *Population Change and Social Planning*. London: Edward Arnold.

Faludi, Susan (1991) *Backlash: The Undeclared War Against Women*. London: Chatto & Windus, London

Family Planning Association (1996) *Contraceptive Choices; Supporting Effective Use of Methods*. London: Family Planning Association.

Family Policy Studies Centre (1990) *Family Changes*. London: FPSC.

Findlay, Allen and Findlay, Anne (1987) *Population and Development in the Third World*. London: Methuen.

Firestone, Shulamith (1970) *The Dialectic of Sex: The Case for Feminist Revolution*. New York: William Morrow.

Fisher, Berenice (1992) 'Against the grain: lives of women without children', *Iris*, **12** (2, Spring/Summer).

Foster, Peggy (1995) *Women and the Health Care Industry: An Unhealthy Relationship?*. Buckingham: Open University Press.

Fox, Nicholas J. (1993) *Postmodernism, Sociology and Health*. Buckinghan: Open University Press.

Freud, Sigmund (1905) 'Three essays on the theory of sexuality', in *On Sexuality* (1977). Harmondsworth: Penguin.

Freud, Sigmund (1932) 'Femininity, Lecture xxxiii', in James Strachery (1964) *New Introductory Lectures on Psycho-Analysis and Other Works*. London: Hogerth Press.

Friday, Nancy (1979) *My Mother, My Self*. London: Fontana.

Friedan, Betty (1963) *The Feminine Mystique*. London: Gollancz.

Fromer, Margot Joan (1983) *Ethical Issues in Sexuality and Reproduction*. Missouri: The C. V. Mosby Company.

Fryer, Peter (1965) *The Birth Controllers*. London: Secker and Warburg.

Gamman, Lorraine and Marshment, Margaret (eds) (1988) *The Female Gaze*. London: Women's Press.

Garcia, Jo, Kilpatrick, Robert, and Richards, Martin (eds) *The Politics of Maternity Care: Services for Childbearing Women in Twentieth-Century Britain*. Oxford: Oxford University Press.

Gavron, Hannah (1966) *The Captive Wife: Conflicts of Housebound Mothers*. London: Penguin.

Gergen, Mary McCanney (ed.) (1988) *Feminist Thought and the Structure of Knowledge*. New York: New York University Press.

Giddens, Anthony (1987) *Social Theory and Modern Sociology*. Cambridge: Polity Press.

Gilman, Charlotte Perkins (1911) *The Man-Made World or Our Androcentric Culture*. London: T. Fisher Unwin.

Glenn, Evelyn Nakano, Chang, Grace and Forcey, Linda Rennie (eds) (1994) *Mothering: Ideology, Experience and Agency*. London: Routledge.

Goldberg, Steven (1979) *Male Dominance: The Inevitability of Patriarchy*. London: Abacus Sphere Books.

Goldscheider, C. (ed.) *Fertility Transitions, Family Structure and Population Policy*. Boulder, CO: Westview Press.

Golombok, Susan and Fivush, Robyn (1994) *Gender Development*. Cambridge: Cambridge University Press.

Gordon, Linda (1976) *Woman's Body, Woman's Rights: A Social History of Birth Control in America*. New York: Grossman.

Gordon, Tuula (1990) *Feminist Mothers*. London: Macmillan.

Graham, H. (1984) *Women, Health and the Family*. London: Harvester Wheatsheaf.

Graham-Smith, Francis (ed.) (1994) *Population, the Complex Reality: A Report of the Population Summit of the World's Scientific Academics*. London: The Royal Society.

Grant, Linda (1993) *Sexing the Millennium: A Political History of the Sexual Revolution*. London: Harper Collins.

Greer, Germaine (1970) *The Female Eunuch*. London: MacGibbon and Kee.

Greer, Germaine (1984) *Sex and Destiny*. London: Secker and Warburg.

Grubacker, Marianne (1988) *There's a Good Girl*. London: Women's Press.

Guardian (1993) 'No kids on the block', 11 April 1995.

Guardian 'World heads for disaster', 28 Jan. 1997.

Guardian (1997) 'Avoiding the bitter morning-after pill', 18 March 1997.

Hanmer, Jalna (1993) 'Women and reproduction', in D. Richardson and V. Robinson (eds) *Introducing Women's Studies*. Basingstoke: Macmillan.

Hannisch, Carol (1971) 'The personal is political', in J. Agel (ed.) *The Radical Therapist*. New York: Ballantine.

Hart, Nicky (1985) *The Sociology of Health and Medicine*. Lancs: Causeway Press.

Hartmann, Heidi (1981). 'The unhappy marriage of Marxism and Feminism: towards a more progressive union', in L. Sargent (ed.) *Women and Revolution: A Discussion of the Unhappy Marriage of Marxism and Feminism*. Boston, MA: South End Press.

Hill, Bridget (1989) *Women, Work, and Sexual Politics in Eighteenth-Century England*. Oxford: Basil Blackwell.

Himes, Norman E. (ed.) (1963) *Medical History of Contraception*. New York: Gamut Press.

Hoffer, Peter C. and Hull, N. E. H. (1981) *Murdering Mothers: Infanticide in England and New England 1558–1803*. New York: New York University School of Law.

Hollway, Wendy (1989) *Subjectivity and Method in Psychology: Gender, Meaning, and Science*. London: Sage.

Homans, Hilary (ed.) (1985) *The Sexual Politics of Reproduction*. Hants: Gower.

Honderich, Ted (ed.) (1995) *The Oxford Companion to Philosophy*. Oxford: Oxford University Press.

hooks, bell (1982) *ain't I a woman? Black Women and Feminism*. London: Pluto Press.

Horney, Karen (1967) *Feminine Psychology*. New York: W. W. Norton.

Hufnagel, Vicki (1990) *No More Hysterectomies*. Northants: Thorsons Publishers Ltd.

Humm, Maggie (1989) *The Dictionary of Feminist Theory*. London: Harvester Wheatsheaf.

Hunt, Sheila and Symonds, Anthea (1995) *The Social Meaning of Midwifery*. London: Macmillan.

Hunt, Sheila and Symonds, Anthea (1996) *The Midwife and Society: Perspectives, Policies and Practice*. London: Macmillan.

Huston, Perdita (1992) *The Right to Choose: Pioneers in Women's Health and Family Planning*. London: Earthscan Publications Ltd.

Hutter, Bridget and Williams, Gillian (eds) (1981) *Controlling Women: The Normal and the Deviant*. London: Croom Helm.

International Planned Parenthood Federation (ed. Ronald L. Kleinman) (1980) *Family Planning Handbook for Doctors*. London: IPPF Medical Publications.

Irigaray, Luce (1985) *This Sex which is not One* (trans.) (1977, *Ce sexe qui nen pas est un*). New York: Cornell University Press.

Jackson, Margaret (1994) *The Real Facts of Life: Feminism, and the Politics of Sexuality*. London: Taylor and Francis.

Jackson, Stevi (1992) 'Women and the family', in Richardson and Robinson (eds) (1993) *Introducing Women's Studies*. London: Macmillan.

Jackson, Stevi *et al.* (eds) (1993) *Women's Studies: A Reader*. London: Harvester Wheatsheaf.

Jacobson, Jodie L. (1990) 'The global politics of abortion', *Worldwatch*, Paper 97 (July). Washington DC.

Jeffreys, Sheila (1985) *The Spinster and Her Enemies*. London: Pandora Press.

Johnson, Stanley P. (1994) *World Population: Turning the Tide. Three Decades of Progress*. London: Graham and Trotman Ltd.

Kaplan, Meryle Mahrer (1992) *Mothers' Images of Motherhood*. London: Routledge.

Kessell, Elton and Mumford, Stephen (1982) 'Potential demand for voluntary female sterilization in the 1980s: the compelling need for a non-surgical method', *Fertility and Sterility* (June 1982).

Klein, R. D. (1983) *Infertility: Women Speak Out about their Experiences of Reproductive Medicine*. London: Pandora.

Klitsch, Michael (1982) 'Sterilization without surgery', *International Family Planning Perspective*, 8, (3, September).

Knowlton, Charles (1841) *The Fruits of Philosophy, or The Private Companion of Young Married People*. London: Freethought Publishing Company.

Lanson, Lucienne (1975) *From Woman to Woman: A Gynaecologist Answers Questions about You and Your Body*. Hermondsworth: Penguin Books.

Leap, Nicky and Hunter, Billie (1993) *The Midwife's Tale: An Oral History from Handywoman to Professional Midwife*. London: Scarlett Press.

Leathard, Audrey (1980) *The Fight for Family Planning*. London: Macmillan.

Lees, Sue (1986) *Losing Out*. London: Hutchinson.

Leonard Barker, Diana and Allen, Sheila (eds) (1976) *Sexual Divisions and Society: Process and Change*. London: Taristock.

Leroy, Margaret (1988) *Miscarriage*. London: Macmillan.

Letherby, Gayle (1994) 'Mother or not, mother or what?: problems of definition and identity', *Women's Studies International Forum*, 17 (5) 525–32.

Letherby, Gayle (1997) ' "Infertility" and "involuntary childlessness": definition and self-identity'. Unpublished PhD thesis, Staffordshire University.

LeVay, Simon (1993) *The Sexual Brain*. Oxford: Basil Blackwell.

Lewis, M. and Rosenblum, L. A. (eds) (1979) *The Child and its Family*. New York: Plenum.

Lovell, Terry (ed.) (1990) *British Feminist Thought*. Oxford: Basil Blackwell.

Lyman, Karen A. (1996) 'Infantilization: the medical model of care', in Phil Brown (ed.) *Perspectives in Medical Sociology*. Illinois: Waveland Press.

McAllister, Fiona with Clarke, Lynda (1998) *Choosing Childlessness*. London: Family Policy Studies Centre.

McCormack, Thelma (1989) 'When is biology destiny?', in Christine Overall (ed.), *The Future of Human Reproduction*. Toronto: Woman's Press.

McLeod, Eileen (1994) *Women's Experience of Feminist Therapy and Counselling*. Buckingham: Open University Press.

McLeod, John (1994) *An Introduction to Counselling*. Buckingham: Open University Press.

Maddox, Brenda (1991) *The Pope and Contraception: The Diabolical Doctrine*. Chatto Counter Blasts No. 18; London: Chatto and Windus.

Madoc-Jones, Beryl and Coates, Jennifer (eds) (1996) *An Introduction to Women's Studies*. Oxford: Blackwell.

Maine, Deborah *et al.* (1995) 'Risks and rights: the uses of reproductive health data', *Reproductive Health Matters* 6, (November), 40–52.

Mamdani, Mahmood (1972) *The Myth of Population Control: Family, Caste and Class in an Indian Village*. London and New York: Monthly Review Press.

Marshall, Helen (1993) *Not Having Children*. Australia: OUP.

Martin, Emily (1989) *The Woman in the Body*. Milton Keynes: Open University Press.

Mass-Observation (1945) 'Britain and her birth-rate: a report prepared for the Advertising Services Guild'. London: John Murray.

Maynard, Mary and Purvis, June (1994) *Researching Women's Lives from a Feminist Perspective*. London: Taylor and Francis.

Mead, Margaret (1935) *Sex and Temperament in Three Primitive Societies*. New York: William Morrow.

Mead, Margaret (1949) *Male and Female: A Study of the Sexes in a Changing World*. New York: (reprinted Penguin, 1971) Dell.

Midwifery Digest (1997) 7, (4, December).

Mies, Marie (1983) 'Towards a methodology for feminist research', in Bowles and Duelli Klein (eds), *Theories of Women's Studies*. London: Routledge and Kegan Paul.

Miller, Jean Baker (1976) *Towards a New Psychology of Women*. Harmondsworth: Penguin.

Millett, Kate (1970) *Sexual Politics*. New York: Doubleday.

Mitchell, Juliet (1966) 'Women: the longest revolution', *New Left Review*, 40, (reprinted 1984). London: Virago.

Mitchell, Juliet (1971) *Women's Estate*. New York: Pantheon.

Mitchell, Juliet (1974) *Psychoanalysis and Feminism*. London: Allen Lane.

Mitchell, Juliet and Rose, Jacqueline (eds) (1982) *Feminine Sexuality: Jacques Lacan and the Ecole Freudienne*. London: Macmillan.

Moir, A. and Jessell, D. (1989) *Brain Sex: The Real Difference Between Men and Women*. London: Michael Joseph.

Money, J. and Ehrhardt, A. (1972) *Man and Woman, Boy and Girl*. Baltimore Maryland: Johns Hopkins UP.

Morell, Carolyn (1994) *Unwomanly Conduct: The Challenges of Intentional Childlessness*. London: Routledge.

Morris, Jenny (ed.) (1992) *Alone Together: Voices of Single Mothers*. London: Women's Press.

Morris, Professor Simon Conway (1996) 'Staring into the abyss', *Royal Institution Christmas Lectures*, BBC2 (28 Dec.).

National Association of Nurses for Contraception and Sexual Health (1996) 'Nearly one million women at risk of unplanned pregnancy', in *Family Planning Association Contraceptive Education Bulletin* (Autumn), FPA Contraceptive Education Service.

New Internationalist (1985) *Women: A World Report*. London: Methuen.

Newton, John (1982) *The Changing Pattern of Male and Female Sterilisation*. London: Birth Control Trust.

Ni Bhrolchain, M. (ed.) (1994) *New Perspectives on Fertility in Britain*. OPCS Studies on Medical and Population Subjects, no.55. London: HMSO.

Nice, Vivien E. (1992) *Mothers and Daughters: The Distortion of a Relationship*. London: Macmillan.

Nicholson, Linda (ed.) (1990) *Feminism/Postmodernism*. London: Routledge.

Nicolson, Paula and Ussher, Jane (eds) (1992) *The Psychology of Women's Health and Health Care*. London: Macmillan.

Oakley, Ann (1974) *The Sociology of Housework*. Oxford: Martin Robertson.

Oakley, Ann (1979a) *Becoming a Mother*. Oxford: Martin Robertson.

Oakley, Ann (1979b) *From Here to Maternity*. Middlesex: Penguin Books.

Oakley, Ann (1980) *Women Confined: Towards a Sociology of Childbirth*. London: Martin Robertson.

Oakley, Ann (1981a) *Subject Women*. London: Martin Robertson.

Oakley, Ann (1981b) 'Interviewing women: a contradiction in terms', in Helen Roberts (ed.) *Doing Feminist Research*. London: Routledge.

Oakley, Anne (1984) *Taking it Like a Woman*. London: Fontana.

Oakley, Ann (1990) *Housewife*. London: Penguin.

O'Brien, Mary (1981) *The Politics of Reproduction*. London: Routledge and Kegan Paul.

O'Brien, Mary (1989) *Reproducing the World: Essays in Feminist Theory*. Boulder, Colorado: Westview Press.

Observer (1995) 'New breed of non-parents turns back on family way', 16 April 1995.

Office for National Statistics (1997) *Birth Statistics 1995*. London: HMSO.

Overall, Christine (ed.) (1989) *The Future of Human Reproduction*. Toronto: The Women's Press.

Oxford Women's Health Action Group (1984) *Whose Choice: What Women have to Say about Contraception*. London: Oxford Women's Health Action Group.

Panos (1994) *Private Decisions, Public Debate: Women, Reproduction and Population*. London: Panos Publications Ltd.

Pateman, Carole (1988) *The Sexual Contract*. Cambridge: Polity Press.

Peck, Ellen (1973) *The Baby Trap: An Outspoken Attack on the Motherhood Myth!* London: Heinrich Hanau Publications.

Perry, Janet (1993) *Counselling for Women*. Buckingham: Open University Press.

Petchesky, Rosalind (1980) 'Reproductive freedom: beyond "A woman's right to choose" ', *Signs*, 5, (4), 661–85.

Petchesky, Rosalind Pollack (1995) 'From population control to reproductive rights: feminist fault lines', *Reproductive Health Matters*, 6 (November), 152–62.

Phoenix, Ann (1991) *Young Mothers?* Cambridge: Polity Press.

Phoenix, A., Woollet, A. and Lloyd, E. (eds) (1991) *Motherhood: Meanings, Practices and Ideologies*. London: Sage.

Pollack, Scarlett (1985) 'Sex and the contraceptive act', in Hilary Homans (eds.), *The Sexual Politics of Reproduction*. Hants: Gower.

Price, Jane (1988) *Motherhood: What it Does to Your Mind*. London: Pandora.

Ramazanoglu, Caroline (1988) *Feminisms and the Contradictions of Oppression*. London: Routledge.

Ravindran, T. K. Sundari (1995) 'Women's health policies: organising for change', *Reproductive Health Matters*, 6 (November) 7–11.

Reed, Evelyn and Moriarty, Claire (1973) *Abortion and the Catholic Church: Two Women Defend Women's Rights*. New York: Pathfinder Press.

Reinharz, S. (1983) 'Experiential analysis: a contribution to feminist research', in Bowles and Duelli Klein (eds.), *Theories of Women's Studies*. London: Routledge and Kegan Paul.

Rich, Adrienne (1976) *Of Woman Born: Motherhood as Experience and Institution*. New York: W. W. Norton.

Rich, Adrienne (1979) *On Lies, Secrets and Silence*. New York: W. W. Norton.

Rich, Adrienne (1980) 'Compulsory heterosexuality and lesbian existence', *Signs*, 5 (4), 631–60.

Richardson, Diane (1993) *Women, Motherhood and Childrearing*. London: Macmillan.

Richardson, Diane and Robinson, Victoria (eds) (1993) *Introducing Women's Studies*. London: Macmillan.

Richardson, Laurel (1988) *The Dynamics of Sex and Gender: A Sociological Perspective*. New York: Harper and Row.

Riddick, Ruth (1990) *The Right to Choose: Questions of Feminist Morality*. Dublin: Attic Press.

Roberts, Helen (ed.) (1981a) *Doing Feminist Research*. London: Routledge.

Roberts, Helen (ed.) (1981b) *Women, Health and Reproduction*. London: Routledge.

Roberts, Helen (1990) *Women's Health Counts*. London: Routledge.

Roberts, Helen (1992) *Women's Health Matters*. London: Routledge.

Rose, June (1992) *Marie Stopes and the Sexual Revolution*. London: Faber and Faber.

Rowbotham, Sheila (1972) *Women, Resistance and Revolution*. Harmondsworth: Penguin.

Rowbotham, Sheila (1973) *Hidden From History: 300 Years of Women's Oppression and the Fight Against It*. London: Pluto.

Rowbotham, Sheila (1977) *Woman's Consciousness, Man's World*. London: Pelican.

Rowbotham, Sheila (1981) 'To be or not to be: the dilemma of mothering', *Feminist Review*, 39, 82–91.

Rowland, Robyn (1992) *Living Laboratories: Women and Reproductive Technology*. London: Cedar.

Ruddick, Sara (1982) 'Maternal thinking' in B. Thorne and M. Yalom (eds) *Rethinking the Family: Some Feminist Questions*. London: Longman.

Russell, Diana (1989) *Lives of Courage: Women For a New South Africa*. New York: Basic Books.

Sanger, Margaret (1920) *Woman and the New Race*. USA: Truth Publishing Company.

Sanger, Margaret (1932) *My Fight for Birth Control*. London: Faber and Faber.

Savage, Wendy (1986) *A Savage Enquiry: Who Controls Childbirth?* London: Virago. London

Sayers, Janet (1982) *Biological Politics: Feminist and Anti-Feminist Perspectives*. London: Tavistock.

Scambler, Graham (ed.) (1991) (3rd edn.) *Sociology as Applied to Medicine*. London: Bailliere Tindal.

Scully, Diana (1980) *Men Who Control Women's Health: The Miseducation of Obstetrician–Gynecologists*. Boston: Houghton Mifflin Company.

Seal, Vivien (1990) *Whose Choice? Working-Class Women and the Control of Fertility*. London: Fortress Books.

Seale, Clive and Pattison, Stephen (eds) (1994) (2nd edn) *Medical Knowledge: Doubt and Certainty*. Buckingham: Open University Press.

Shakin, M., Shakin, D. and Sternglanz, S. H. (1985) 'Infant clothing: sex labelling for strangers', *Sex Roles*. **12**, 955–63.

Shallatt, Lezak (1995) 'Business as usual for quinacrine sterilisation in Chile', *Reproductive Health Matters*, **6** (November), 144–7.

Sharpe, Sue (1976) *Just Like a Girl: How Girls Learn to be Women*. Harmondsworth: Penguin.

Sherwin, Susan (1989) 'Feminist ethics and new reproductive technologies', in Christine Overall (ed.) *The Future of Human Reproduction*. Toronto: Women's Press.

Shilling, Chris (1993) *The Body and Social Theory*. London: Sage Publication.

Shotter, John and Logan, Josephine (1988) 'The pervasiveness of patriarchy: on finding a different voice', in *Feminist Thought and the Structure of Knowledge* (Mary McCanney Gergen (ed.)). New York: New York UP.

Siann, Gerda (1994) *Gender Sex and Sexuality: Contemporary Psychological Perspectives*. London: Taylor & Francis.

Simms, Madeleine (1985) 'Legal abortion in Great Britain', in Hilary Homans (ed.), *The Sexual Politics of Reproduction*. Hants: Gower.

Skevington, S. and Baker, D. (1984) *Women, and Self-Identity*. London: Sage.

Skevington, S. and Baker, D. (eds) (1989) *The Social Identity of Women*. London: Sage.

Smart, Carol (1984) *The Ties That Bind: Marriage and the Reproduction of Patriarchal Relations*. London: Routledge.

Smart, Carol (1992) *Regulating Motherhood: Historical Essays on Marriage, Motherhood and Sexuality*. London: Routledge.

Spender, Dale (ed.) (1983) *Feminist Theorists: Three Centuries of Women's Intellectual Traditions*. London: The Women's Press.

Stacey, Margaret (1988) *The Sociology of Health and Healing: A Textbook*. London: Unwin Hyman.

Stanley, Liz and Wise, Sue (1983) 'Back into the personal, or our attempt to construct feminist research', in Bowles and Duelli Klein (eds) *Theories of Women's Studies*. London: Routledge and Kegan Paul.

Stanley, L. and Wise, A (1988) *Breaking Out Again: Feminist Ontology and Epistemology*. London: Routledge.

Stein, Dorothy (1995) *People Who Count: Population and Politics, Women and Children*. London: Earthscan Publications Ltd.

Stopes, Marie Carmichael (1918) *Married Love: A New Contribution to the Solution of Sexual Difficulties*. London: G. P. Putnam's Sons.

Stopes, Marie Carmichael (1918) *Wise Parenthood: A Practical Sequel to 'Married Love'*. London: G. P. Putnam's Sons.

Stopes, Marie Carmichael (1920) *Radiant Motherhood: A Book for those who are Creating the Future*. London: G. P. Putnam's Sons.

Stopes, Marie Carmichael (1923) *Contraception (Birth Control): Its Theory, History and Practice, A Manual for Medical and Legal Professions*. London: G. P. Putnam's Sons.

Stopes, Marie Carmichael (1926) *The Human Body*. London: The Gill Publishing Co Ltd.

Strachey, James (1964) *Sigmund Freud: New Introductory Lectures on Psycho-Analysis and Other Works*. London: The Hogarth Press.

Sunday Pictorial (1949) 'Homes without babies' 1949 (undated). Archive, University of Sussex in Brighton: Mass-Observation Archive.

The Sunday Times (1995) 'Mum's not the word', 16 April 1995.

Sydie, R. A. (1987) *Natural Women, Cultured Men: A Feminist Perspective on Sociological Theory*. Milton Keynes: Open University Press.

Taylor, Timothy (1996) *The Prehistory of Sex: Four Million Years of Human Sexual Culture*. London: Fourth Estate.

Tong, Rosemarie (1989) *Feminist Thought: A Comprehensive Introduction*. London: Unwin Hyman.

Trebilcot, Joyce (ed.) (1983) *Mothering: Essays in Feminist Theory*. Washington; Maryland: Rowland & Littlefield Publishers.

Turner, Bryan S. (1987) *Medical Power and Social Knowledge*. London: Sage.

Turner, Lyn (1993) 'Risk and contraception: what women are not told about tubal ligation', *Women's Studies International Forum*, **16** (5), 471–86.

UN Chronicle (September 1994) 'Population. Choices and responsibilities: finding the balance'. United Nations Department of Public Information, **31** (3), 40–3.

UN Chronicle (September 1994) 'Population. Reproductive rights, family planning: a cornerstone of control'. United Nations Department of Public Information, **31** (3), 46.

UN Chronicle (September 1994) 'Seeking equality. Empowering women: an essential objective'. United Nations Department of Public Information, **31** (3), 47.

UN Chronicle (December 1994) 'Population and development. Cairo conference reaches consensus on plan to stabilize world growth by 2015: the 20-year programme of action'. United Nations Department of Public Information, **31** (4).

UNFPA (1997) *The State of World Population 1997. The Right to Choose: Reproductive Rights and Reproductive Health*. United Nations Family Planning Association.

Unger, R. K. (1979) 'Towards a redefinition of sex and gender', *American Psychologist*, **34**, 1085–94.

Valverde, M. (1985) *Sex, Power, and Pleasure*. Toronto: Women's Press.

Veevers, Jean (1980) *Childless By Choice*. Ontario: Butterworth.

Walby, Sylvia. (1990) *Theorizing Patriarchy*. Oxford: Basil Blackwell.

Walker, Moira (1990) *Women in Therapy and Counselling*. Buckingham: Open University Press.

Walkerdine, Valerie (1989) *Counting Girls Out*. London: Virago Press.

Walkerdine, Valerie and Lucey, Helen (1989) *Democracy in the Kitchen: Regulating Mothers and Socialising Daughters*. London: Virago.

Wandor, Michelene (ed.) (1972) *The Body Politic: Women's Liberation in Britain 1969–1972*. London: Stage 1.

Warnock, Mary (1984) *A Question of Life*. Oxford: Basil Blackwell.

Webb, C. (1986) *Feminist Practice in Women's Health Care*. Chichester: John Wiley & Sons.

Webster, Richard (1996) *Why Freud Was Wrong: Sin, Science and Psychoanalysis*. London: Fontana Press (Harper Collins).

Weedon, Chris (1987) *Feminist Practice and Poststructuralist Theory*. New York: Basil Blackwell.

Weiner, Gaby (ed.) (1985) *Just a Bunch of Girls; Feminist Approaches to Schooling*. Milton Keynes: Open University Press.

Wilkinson, Sue and Kitzinger, Celia (eds) (1993) *Heterosexuality*. London: Sage.

Wilkinson, Sue and Kitzinger, Celia (eds) (1994) *Women and Health: Feminist Perspectives*. London: Taylor & Francis.

Winn, Denise (1988) *Experiences of Abortion*. London: Macdonald and Co.

Winston, R. M. L. (1977) 'Why 103 women asked for reversal of sterilisation', *British Medical Journal*, 2 (30 July 1977), 305–7.

Wollstonecraft, Mary (1992) (1792) *A Vindication of the Rights of Women*. London: Penguin Classics.

Women's Health Journal (1997) February, 2.

Wood, Clive (1974) *Vasectomy and Sterilization: A Guide For Men and Women*. London: Maurice Temple Smith.

Wood, Clive and Suitters, Beryl (1970) *The Fight for Acceptance: A History of Contraception*. Aylesbury: Medical and Technical Publishing Co. Ltd.

Wood, Julia (1994) *Gendered Lives: Communication, Gender, and Culture*. California: Wadsworth Publishing Company.

Worell, Judith and Remer, Pam (1992) *Feminist Perspectives in Therapy: An Empowerment Model for Women*. Chichester: John Wiley & Sons Ltd.

Wylie, Evan McLeod (1972) *A Guide to Voluntary Sterilization: The New Birth Control*. USA: Grossett and Dunlap.

Yalom, I. D., Green, R. and Fisk, N. (1973) 'Prenatal exposure to female hormones', *Archives of General Psychiatry*, 28, 554–61.

Index

costs of sterilization and reversal 113, 126–7
counselling 122, 126, 136–9, 148
  inconsistent use of term 37, 137
  lack of, cause for concern 137–9
  as positive and worthwhile experience 138
  as 'stalling' tactic 137
counsellors' suspicions about childfree 133
couples without children 2, 6
creationist belief 48

Darwin, Charles 59
decisions 2, 6, 86, 90–1, 106, 134
  childfree and sterilization years apart 94, 162
  childfree decisions wrong 87
  couples, on sterilization 6, 8, 76, 109
  people taking final responsibility for lives 152
  reproductive 116
decreasing population warnings 1, 53–4
delays, medical 119, 125
'delay-time' 143, 149
desperation to have children 104
  women 110
determination 6, 10, 81–2, 114, 122–4, 136, 139, 141–3, 158, 162
'deviant', non–mothering women 47, 100
  women's sexual freedom 48
diaries 16–33
diary writing 8, 10–13
difference of opinion, medical 119
differences, between
  childfree and childless 117, 141, 157
  childfree sterilized and childfree 'postponers' 4–6, 89–90, 159–60
  childfree and women with children 5, 47, 161
  sterilized childfree and sterilized mothers 82, 124, 129
different choices by childfree women 5, 9
disability and challenges, women's voice 9
disapproval of childfree 38, 98
  by GPs and consultants 6, 79, 128, 152–3
dissatisfaction, available contraception 3, 36, 75, 91–4, 113, 141–2, 147
divisions between women 82, 104, 152
double-standards (between women and men) 48

dread of getting pregnant 63
drop in family size 57

ectopic pregnancy 79, 146
education of girls 40
Eilbeck, Chris ('Getting off the reproductive bicycle') 111
elective sterilization 3–5, 6, 15, 37–8, 49, 83, 162–3
emotions 11, 114
empowerment through reproductive control 69, 115
'English race' 58
envy of childfree 106
ethics, GPs and consultants 122, 131
eugenics 9, 35, 59–60, 118
  supporters 59
Eugenics Society 59

failed contraception 77, 105
  women's experiences 16–33, 87–9, 105
failure rates
  of contraception
  of sterilization 79–80
family 57, 66, 72, 96–8, 162
  black women's criticism of feminist critique 97
  'cereal-box' image 97
  as 'site of gender struggle' 96
  size, changes in attitudes 57
Family Planning Association 90, 113
Family Policy Studies Centre 1, 54, 90
fear of pregnancy 93
feminist research methods 7–10, 33
feminists 38 n. 2, 114
'feminization of poverty' 71
fertility control 114
  cultural restrictions 67
  by medical profession 3, 118
  as unresolved issue for women 35, 49
  by women 1, 49, 61, 63–5, 83, 87, 157
  of women by men 64
final choice 2, 162
  sterilization too final 89–9, 138
'friendship wedges' 104

gatekeepers, GPs and other medics as 128–30, 150
  cautious guidelines for 130
gender
  ascribed at birth 41
  biological theories 42 (*see also* sociobiology)